FUNDAMENTALS

OF

CARDIOLOGY

CONCISE REVIEW BOOK FOR

USMLE STEP 1-2-3 AND GENERAL MEDICAL BOARDS

SECOND EDITION, 2016

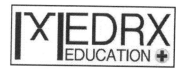

www.medrx-education.com

BY

CHIRAG NAVADIA, MD

INTRODUCTION

Hello friends,

I am glad to present second edition of renowned clinical review book 'Fundamentals of Cardiology' for USMLE and other general clinical purposes. This book mainly focuses on fundamental clinical concepts of USMLE step 1-3, ABFM and ABIM exam. Book begins with high yield general concepts of anatomy and physiology that will be helpful to any new learner.

After reviewing few preclinical chapters, the real fun of cardiovascular medicine begins. This section primarily provides with up-to-date and most recent information on various etiologies, mechanisms, clinical associations, investigation of choice, and primary managements about each and every high yield cardiology topics. This will help you to score some extra points on your Step 2-3 and family medicine/internal medicine board exams.

Most of the investigations and managements are referred from reputed cardiology resources, which make this book accurate and reliable. Each and every information is incorporated in best possible way to make this book an easy learning guide for students, interns, nurses, and even general physician.

"THUNDERNOTE" is a new concept that we adapted for this book. Thunder-notes are detailed side-notes that connect you with the relevant topic of a different subject and thus allow to review another clinical resource. At the end, there is a brief summary of cardiac pharmacology, which describes each drug with its mechanism and common side effects.

I want you to finish this book with smiling face ☺. A full refund awaits any reader of this book that did not like it or feels the content he wanted to review is not covered in this book (14-days full money back guarantee). If you can give me your two minutes, please give a good and honest rating on Amazon.

Sincerely,

CHIRAG NAVADIA, MD

Founder of medrx-education.com

DISCLAIMER

All printed and/or digital content is for educational and/or learning use only. We are not responsible for the utilization of any knowledge, information or facts gained from the printed and/or digital content in the practice of medicine, medical research or any related medical or science applications.

Also, while materials available in this book may be useful for medical coursework examinations and qualifying examinations such as the NCLEX™, USMLE™, ABFM™, and ABIM™. You understand that MEDRX is not by any means affiliated with any other third party. Moreover, it is not (directly or by implication) giving any guarantees that the materials provided by us are tested on these examinations.

Of all the investigations and management mentioned in this book, almost 95% are based upon guidelines that were released by American Heart Association between 2010-2014. However, you realize that errors can occur, and thus administrators that we referred to in this book should not be used directly in clinical practice without any guidance. We are not responsible for any harm is done to anybody by the administrators described in this book.

Certain images were freely available on the internet, and we had adapted them with full credits. We have permissions to use most of the pictures that are available in this book. However, we were unable to reach all publishers or don't know the real owner in few cases. If anybody have any objection to the image used in this book, feel free to contact us through our website and that particular image will be removed immediately.

Printed in the United States of America

Print number: 0 9 8 7 6 5 4 3 2

About USMLE

The UNITED STATES MEDICAL LICENSING EXAMINATION is a three-step examination for medical licensure in the United States. It is sponsored by Federation of State Medical Boards (FSMB) and the National Board of Medical Examiners (NBME).

Step 1 assesses whether you understand and can apply important concepts of the sciences basic to the practice of medicine, with special emphasis on principles and mechanisms underlying health, disease, and modes of therapy. Step 1 ensures mastery of not only the sciences that provide a foundation for the safe and competent practice of medicine in the present, but also the scientific principles required for maintenance of competence through lifelong learning. Step 1 is constructed according to an integrated content outline that organizes basic science material along two dimensions: Step 1 is a **one-day** examination. It is divided into seven 60-minute blocks and administered in one 8-hour testing session The number of questions per block on a given examination form will vary, but will not exceed 40. The total number of items on the overall examination form will not exceed 280.

Step 2CK assesses whether you can apply medical knowledge, skills, and understanding of clinical science essential for the provision of patient care under supervision and includes emphasis on health promotion and disease prevention. Step 2 ensures that due attention is devoted to principles of clinical sciences and basic patient-centered skills that provide the foundation for the safe and competent practice of medicine. Step 2 CK is a **one-day** examination. It is divided into eight 60-minute blocks, and administered in one 9-hour testing session. The number of items in a block will be displayed at the beginning of each block. This number will vary among blocks, but will not exceed 44 items. Regardless of the number of items, 60 minutes are allotted for the completion of each block.

On the test day for both Step 1 and Step 2CK, examinees have a minimum of 45 minutes of break time and a 15- minute optional tutorial. The amount of time available for breaks may be increased by finishing a block of test items or the optional tutorial before the allotted time expires.

Step 2 CS uses standardized patients to test medical students and graduates on their ability to gather information from patients, perform physical examinations, and communicate their findings to patients and colleagues. Step 2 CS administration will include **twelve patient encounters**. These include a very small number of no-scored patient encounters, which are added for pilot testing new cases and other research purposes. Such cases are not counted in determining your score. You will have **15 minutes** for each and 10-minutes for writing patient's notes.

Step 3 assesses whether you can apply medical knowledge and understanding of biomedical and clinical science essential for the unsupervised practice of medicine, with emphasis on patient management in ambulatory settings. The test items and cases reflect the clinical situations that a general, as-yet undifferentiated, physician might encounter within the context of a specific setting. Step 3 provides a final assessment of physicians assuming independent responsibility for delivering general medical care. Step 3 is a **two-day** examination. The first day of testing includes 233 multiple-choice items divided into 6 blocks of 38-40 items; 60 minutes are allotted for completion of each block of test items. **Items with an associated pharmaceutical advertisement or scientific abstract are included in each of these multiple-choice blocks.** There are approximately 7 hours in the test session on the first day, including 45 minutes of break time and a 5-minute optional tutorial.
There are approximately 9 hours in the test session on the second day. This day of testing includes a 5-minute optional tutorial followed by 180 multiple-choice items, divided into 6 blocks of 30 items; 45 minutes are allotted for completion of each block of test items. The second day also includes a 7-minute CCS tutorial. This is followed by 13 case simulations, each of which is allotted a maximum of 10 or 20 minutes of real time. A minimum of 45 minutes is available for break time.

TABLE OF CONTENTS

- The heart develops from splanchnic mesoderm in the later half of 3rd week and starts beating by the 4th week of gestation. Neural crest cell migration plays a significant role in the development of the heart.

- Single heart tube is formed by the fusion of primordial heart tubes (cardiogenic cells). Heart tube will undergo dextral looping (bend to right), rotation, and other changes that will give rise to various embryological dilations such as truncus arteriosus, bulbus cordis, primitive ventricle, primitive atrium and sinus venosus.

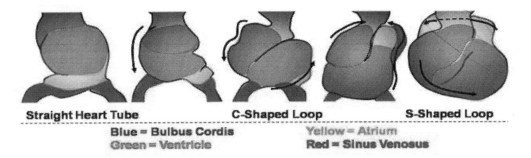

Straight Heart Tube   C-Shaped Loop   S-Shaped Loop

Blue = Bulbus Cordis   Yellow = Atrium
Green = Ventricle   Red = Sinus Venosus

Figure 1.1: sequence of events in embryological development of the heart

EMBRYONIC STRUCTURE	ADULT DERIVATIVE
Truncus arteriosus	Ascending aorta, pulmonary trunk, semilunar valves
Bulbus cordis	Smooth part of left ventricle (aortic vestibule) and right ventricles (conus arteriosus)
Primitive atria	Trabeculated part of atria
Primitive ventricles	Trabeculated part of ventricles
Left horn of sinus venosus	Coronary sinus
Right horn of sinus venosus	Smooth part of right atrium

CLINICAL NOTE: KARTAGENER SYNDROME

Pathogenesis: Defect in dynein arms.

Dynein arms primarily mediate cardiac looping. A defect in these arms will not allow the heart to shift toward left side and therefore, right-sided heart (dextrocardia) is seen in this pathology.

Clinical presentation: Bronchiectasis, chronic sinusitis and situs inversus (in about 50% case only)

Most common infectious organisms: Staphylococcus aureus, Hemophilus influenza, Streptococcus pneumonia

Management: Routine follow-up, treat symptomatically (no guidelines exist due to lack of data)

VASCULAR DEVELOPMENT

Detailed discussion on looping of heart and vascular development is extremely low-yield for any medical personal, however I had decided to highlight few important points that can be tested on usmle step 1 exam.

Development of arterial system:

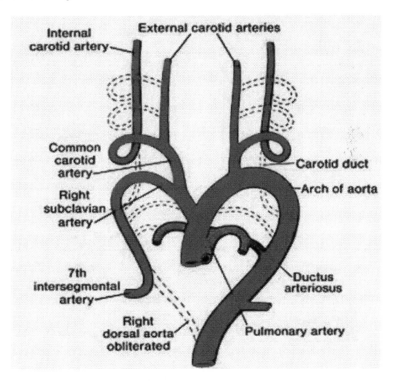

Figure 1.2: aortic arch derivatives

AORTIC ARCH	CRANIAL NERVE	ARTERIAL DERIVATIVE
1st	Trigeminal nerve	Part of maxillary artery (branch of external carotid artery)
2nd	Facial nerve	Stapedial and hyoid artery
3rd	Glossopharyngeal nerve	Common carotid artery and proximal internal carotid artery

4th	Superior branch of vagus nerve	**Right side** - right subclavian artery **Left side** - arch of aorta
5th	-	Obliterates
6th	Vagus nerve (recurrent laryngeal nerve)	**Right side** – proximal pulmonary artery **Left side** - ductus arteriosus

Development of aorta:

- **Ascending aorta** is derived from lateral plate of mesoderm
- **Arch of aorta** is derived from neural crest cells
- **Descending aorta** is derived from paraxial mesoderm (somite)

Development of venous system:

- **Vitelline veins (omphalomesenteric)** will develop into veins of the liver (sinusoids, hepatic portal vein, hepatic vein) and some part of inferior vena cava.

- **Umbilical vein** remnant is known as ligamentum teres of the liver.

- **Cardinal veins** will contribute to larger veins of the body like brachiocephalic, superior vena cava, inferior vena cava, azygos and renal veins.

THUNDERNOTE: SINGLE UMBILICAL ARTERY

- **Single umbilical artery** is the most common umbilical anomaly.
- It can be normal in many cases. However, periodic checkups are required.
- It can be associated with Edward syndrome (trisomy 18).

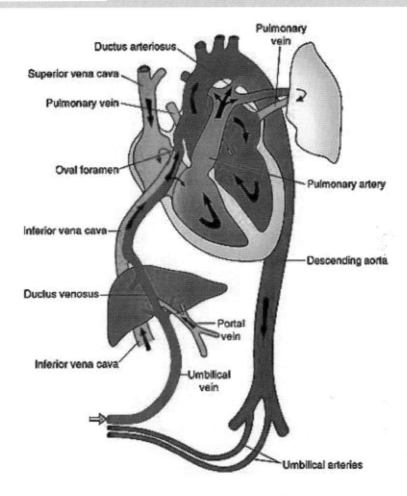

Figure 1.3: fetal blood circulation

Remnants of fetal structure in adult:

- The remnant of the umbilical vein is called ligamentum teres of the liver.

- The remnant of ductus venosus is called ligamentum venosum.

- The remnant of ductus arteriosus is called ligamentum arteriosus (failure to close is called as **patent ductus arteriosus**).

- The remnant of foramen ovale is called as fossa ovalis (patent foramen ovale is normal in many people, **most common causes of paradoxical emboli**).

- The remnant of the umbilical artery is called medial umbilical ligaments.

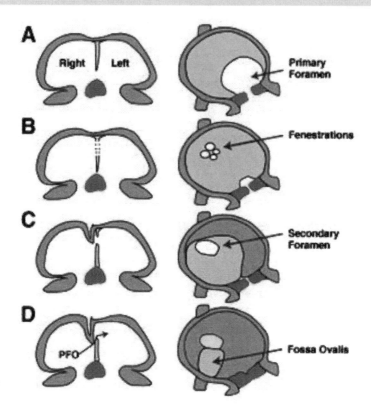

Figure 1.4: septum development of the atrium*

ATRIAL SEPTATION

- **Septum primum** will form in the atrial part of the primitive heart and starts growing toward endocardial cushion. An endocardial cushion is a group of neural crest cells that are migrated to the center of the heart.

- As septum grows downward, **foramen primum** will become narrower, and before foramen primum closes completely, fenestrations will develop in septum primum that forms a hole called as - **foramen secundum.** This foramen is necessary to allow blood flow from right to left side in the fetus.

- After formation of foramen secundum, **septum secundum** starts developing on its right side and will cover most of the foramen secundum. It does not fuse with endocardial cushion and allow some space for flow of blood from the right to left. This space is called as **foramen ovale**.

THUNDERNOTE: PATENT FORAMEN OVALE

- Closure of foramen ovale occurs immediately after the birth due to the decrease in resistance of pulmonary circulation with the first breath of infant. This will increase blood flow to left atrium resulting in high left atrial pressure. This high pressure will close the foramen ovale.

- PFO is a condition in which septum primum and septum secundum fail to fuse after birth. In the beginning, this will lead to a left to right flow of blood. It is an acyanotic condition at the time of birth because a small amount of oxygenated blood from the left atrium will flow back to the right atrium due to the pressure gradient. This oxygenated blood will re-enter pulmonary circulation.

- Over the long period, volume and pressure overload in the pulmonary artery will cause hypertrophy and hyperplasia (pulmonary stenosis like situation) of the pulmonary artery. This will cause an increase in pressure on the right side of the heart resulting in a flow of deoxygenated blood from right atrium to left atrium via foramen ovale. This reversal of blood flow is called as **eissenmenger syndrome.** Thus, the main complication that can develop due to patent foramen ovale is an increased risk of paradoxical emboli.

- **Diagnosis:** transesophageal echocardiography is an investigation of choice in adults with suspected paradoxical emboli.

  Paradoxical emboli triad: raised right atrial pressure, the venous source of thrombosis, and the presence of PFO.

- **Management:** most PFO are left untreated because they usually fuse off later in the life.

  Indication for the closure of PFO: any PFO > 25mm is an indication for surgical closure. Another indication is when a patient develops paradoxical emboli. Give aspirin (in low-risk population) or aspirin + warfarin (in high-risk population) followed by closure of PFO (percutaneous closure or surgically).

VENTRICULAR SEPTATION

- Ventricular septation begins at 4th week and is completed by the end of 7th week.
- **Upper membranous part** of septum arises from the endocardial cushion, conotruncal ridge and grows downward. **Lower muscular part** of septum appears from the floor of ventricles and grows upward.
- The majority of the septum is made up of the muscular part. Failure in the fusion of upper and lower septum will lead to **ventricular septal defect**.
- The endocardial cushion also contributes to the development of all valves and play a significant role for intra-heart partitions. Various neural crest cell abnormalities will affect cardiac septal development.

THUNDERNOTE: NEURAL CREST CELLS ABNORMALITIES

- **Neuroblastoma** (most common extra-cranial tumor in infancy)

- **Di-George syndrome** (due to deletion on chromosome 22, associated with truncus arteriosus and tetralogy of Fallot)

- **Neurofibromatosis type 1** (mutation of neurofibromin gene on chromosome 17)

- **Hirschsprung disease** (aganglionic segment in intestine, baby fails to pass meconium within 48 hours of delivery, part of colon near to anus is usually first to be affected. Definitive diagnosis is made by suction biopsy)

- **Tetralogy of Fallot** (pulmonary stenosis, overriding aorta, ventricular septal defect, and right ventricular hypertrophy)

- **Treacher-Collins syndrome** (congenital disorder with craniofacial deformities like micrognathia, conductive hearing loss, and undeveloped zygoma, mutated gene (TCOF1) act as a precursor of neural crest cell)

- **Melanoma** (tumor of melanocytes, occur due to the DNA damage from UV light, common sites are leg and back, treatment is surgery followed by IL-2 or interferon)

SEPTATION OF TRUNCUS ARTERIOSUS

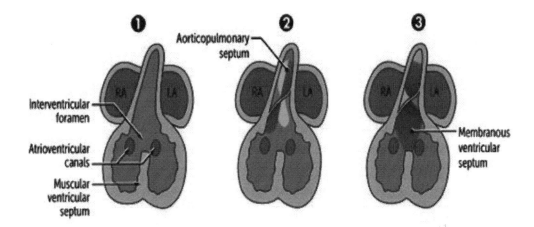

Figure 1.5: septum development in the ventricles and truncus arteriosus*

- Septation of truncus arteriosus will give rise to pulmonary artery and aorta.

Two processes take place in this septation:

1) **Formation of the aortic-pulmonary septum**: the septum will divide truncus arteriosus into two tubes. One tube will form pulmonary artery, and another tube will form aorta.

2) **Spiral rotation:** during the process of septation, initially pulmonary artery is on the left side and aorta is on the right side. Spiral rotation is necessary so that aorta ends up on the left side (to left ventricle) and pulmonary artery ends up on the right side (to the right ventricle).

- Failure of aorticopulmonary septum development will result in **truncus arteriosus** while the failure of spiralization will result in **transposition of great vessels**.

- If aorticopulmonary septum fails to align correctly and shifts anteriorly to right, it will result in tetralogy of Fallot.

MEDIASTINUM

The mediastinum is central, midline thoracic cavity, which is surrounded anteriorly by the sternum, posteriorly by 12 thoracic vertebrae and laterally by pleural cavity.

The mediastinum is divided into the superior mediastinum and inferior mediastinum.

1) Superior mediastinum

- The superior mediastinum is a cavity that is above the plane of sternal angle (above 2nd rib).

- It contains superior vena cava, aortic arch and its branches, trachea, esophagus, thoracic duct, vagus, and phrenic nerve.

2) Inferior mediastinum

- The inferior mediastinum is a cavity that is located below the plane of the sternal angle. It is further divided into three parts - anterior, middle and posterior mediastinum.

  The anterior mediastinum is anterior to the heart and contains remnants of the thymus.

  The middle mediastinum contains the heart and great vessels.

  The posterior mediastinum contains everything that is below the posterior margin of heart i.e. thoracic aorta, esophagus, thoracic duct, azygos veins, and vagus nerve.

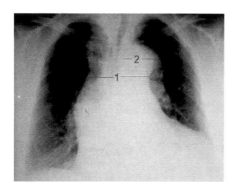

Figure 2.1: Chest x-ray, 1: widened mediastinum, 2: aortic knob*

Widened mediastinum is when the diameter is greater than 6 cm on upright chest x-ray or greater than 8cm on supine chest x-ray. Few causes of widened mediastinum are:

- Aortic dissection
- Dorsal spinal vertebral fracture (T4-T8)
- Infections with bacillus anthracis (anthrax)
- Aortic aneurysm

- Esophageal rupture can present with air in the mediastinum leading to palpable crepitus on the anterior chest wall.

- Most posterior part of the heart is left atrium. The esophagus is located just behind the left atrium. Enlargement of left atrium due to any reasons (most common cause is mitral stenosis) will compress the esophagus, and lead to dysphagia.

- Left atrial enlargement and aortic aneurysm can also cause hoarseness of voice due to compression of the left recurrent laryngeal nerve, which loops around ligamentum arteriosus/arch of the aorta.

- Left vagus nerve branch loops around arch of aorta (right vagus nerve loops around right subclavian artery)

MOST COMMON PATHOLOGY IN MEDIASTINUM

- Most common pathology in anterior mediastinum: **thymoma**

- Most common pathology in middle mediastinum: **congenital cysts**

- Most common pathology in posterior mediastinum: **neurogenic tumors**

- Overall most common pathology in mediastinum: **neurogenic tumors**

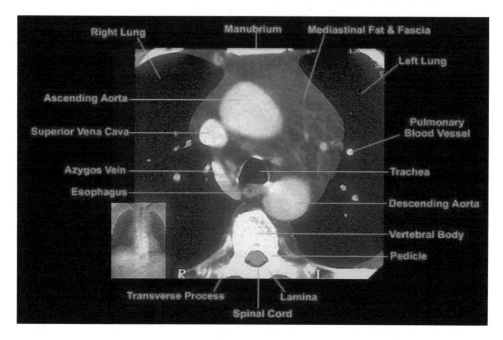

Figure 2.2: CT at T4*

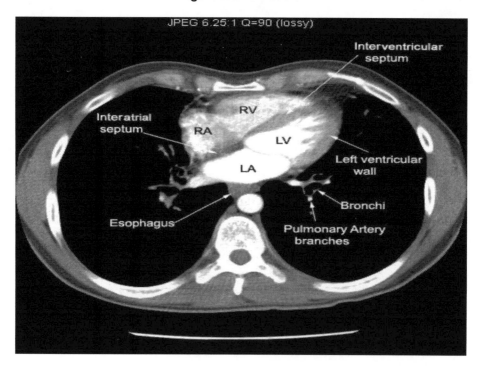

Figure 2.3: CT at T5*

THUNDERNOTE: SUPERIOR VENA CAVA SYNDROME

Superior vena cava syndrome is a group of symptoms that occurs due to external compression of superior vena cava. It is characterized by:

- Shortness of breath
- Facial swelling
- Upper limb edema
- Headache
- Venous distension in head and neck
- Retinal hemorrhage and stroke can also be present

It is a medical emergency because It can raise intracranial pressure and increases risk of aneurysm/rupture of intracranial arteries

It can also compress cervical sympathetic plexus, causing **Horner syndrome**. Horner syndrome is characterized by a classic triad of ipsilateral ptosis, miosis, and anhidrosis.

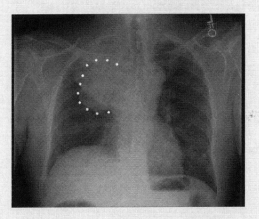

Figure 2.4: mediastinal mass*

Large mediastinal mass that can compress superior vena cava are

- Thymoma
- Burkitt's lymphoma
- Primary lung cancer like small cell carcinoma (most common cause of SVC syndrome)

You cannot distinguish them on chest x-ray. Additional investigations like biopsy are required to confirm the source.

INTERNAL STRUCTURES

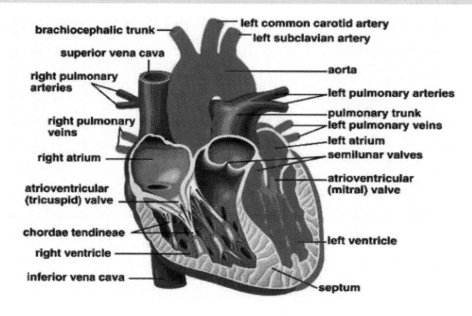

Figure 2.5: internal structures of the heart*

EXTERNAL STRUCTURES

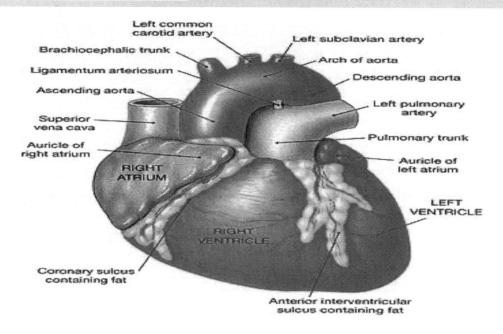

Figure 2.6: external structures of the heart*

FRONTAL VIEW

- The right atrium forms the right border of heart.

- The left ventricle forms the left border of heart on frontal CXR.

- The right ventricle covers the area between the right atrium and left ventricle.

- The left atrium is located posteriorly.

- The apex of the heart is left ventricle.

- The right and left auricles plus conus arteriosus form the superior border while the diaphragm is located inferiorly.

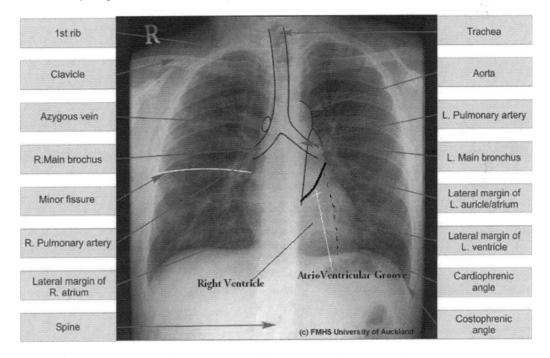

Figure 2.7: frontal view of the chest cavity on chest x-ray*

SURFACE AREA	LOCATION
Upper right	3rd right costal cartilage
Lower right	6th right costal cartilage
Upper left	Inferior margin of 2nd left costal cartilage
Apex of heart	Left 5th intercostal space at midclavicular line

Table 2.1: surface projections of the heart's surface area

BORDER	EXTENSION
Right border	From 3rd right costal cartilage to 6th right costal cartilage
Left border	From 5th left intercostal space at midclavicular line to 2nd left costal cartilage
Inferior border	From 6th right costal cartilage to 5th left intercostal space at midclavicular line
Superior border	From inferior margin of 2nd left costal cartilage to superior margin of 3rd right costal cartilage

Table 2.2: surface projections of the heart's border

Surface projection landmarks of the heart are crucial to remember for 'step 1' exam.

- The right atrium will be pierced by the penetrating injury at the right sternal border at the 4th intercostal space.

- The right ventricle will be pierced by the penetrating injury on the left sternal border at the 4th intercostal space.

- The left ventricle will be pierced by the penetrating injury medial to the left midclavicular line at the 4th intercostal space.

- There is very less likelihood of injury to left atrium due to its posterior location unless a penetrating trauma is deep enough to pass through the upper left side of the heart (bullet injury). In rare instances, dilation of left atrium can compress esophagus posteriorly and cause dysphagia.

THUNDERNOTE: PACEMAKER

A pacemaker is an electronic device that senses electrical heart rhythm and provides electrical stimulation when indicated. There are three approaches that are currently in use:

- **Single chamber pacemaker:** 1 pacing lead is implanted in the right atrium or right ventricles.

- **Dual chamber pacemaker:** 2 pacing leads are inserted (1 in the right ventricle and 1 in the right atrium). This is the most common type of implanted pacemaker.

- **Biventricular pacing (cardiac resynchronization therapy):** Along with the leads in the right atrium and right ventricle, a third lead is advanced from the coronary sinus for left ventricular epicardial pacing. The coronary sinus is located behind the atrioventricular groove.

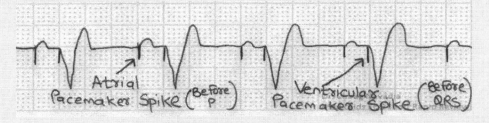

Figure 2.8: atrial and ventricular pacemaker spike*

SKELETAL MUSCLE	CARDIAC MUSCLE	SMOOTH MUSCLE
Striated muscle, actin, and myosin filaments are arranged in sarcomeres	Same as skeletal muscle	Non-striated, more actin than myosin
Well-developed sarcoplasmic reticulum and transverse tubules	Moderately developed	Poorly developed. No transverse tubules
Contains troponin in thin filaments	Same as skeletal muscle	Contain calmodulin (binds to calcium and activates myosin) Nitric oxide (**nitroglycerine**) binds myosin-light chain phosphatase and relaxes venous smooth muscle
Nerve stimulation required for contraction, gap junctions are absent	Action potentials will be generated in **pacemaker** cells and **spreads via gap junctions**	Visceral smooth muscle produces action potentials and current spreads via gap junction

Table 2.3: comparison between cardiac muscle, skeletal muscle and smooth muscle

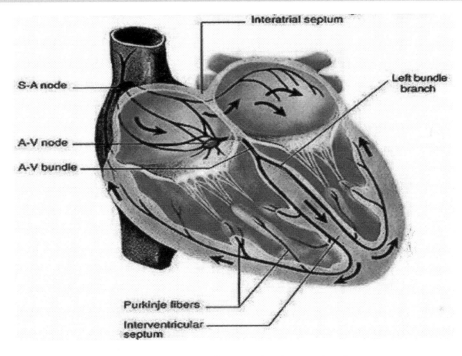

Figure 2.9: cardiac conduction system*

- **Sinoatrial node (SA node)** is a small mass of specialized tissue located in the upper chamber of the right atrium. The sinus node generates an electrical stimulus. This electrical stimulus travels down through the conduction pathways.

- The right and left atria are stimulated first and contract for a short period of time.

- The electrical impulse goes from the SA node to the **atrioventricular node (AV node)**, where impulses are slowed down for a very short period of time and then allowed to continue down the conduction pathway via an electrical channel called the **Bundle of His.**

- The bundle of His divides into right and left pathways to provide electrical stimulation to the right and left ventricles. This causes ventricles to contract and pump out blood to systemic circulation. Each contraction of the ventricles represents one heartbeat.

- **Speed of conduction:** Purkinje > Atria > Ventricles > AV node

- **Pacemakers rhythm generation:** SA (60-100/min) > AV (40-60/min) > bundle of His/Purkinje (20-40/min).

- **Pacemaker cells** uses calcium to generate an action potential. Atrial and ventricular muscle depolarization are sodium-dependent.

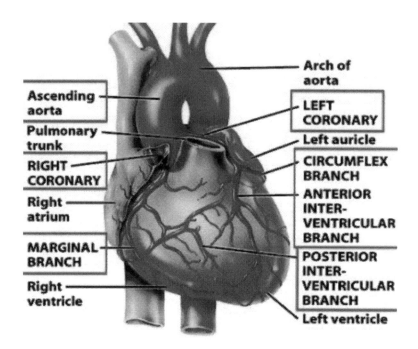

Figure 2.10: territories of coronary arteries*

The heart is supplied by coronary arteries, which arises from the aortic valve.

- The left coronary artery divides into left circumflex artery and left anterior descending artery aka anterior interventricular branch.

  Left circumflex artery supply blood to lateral wall of left ventricle, left atrium and left posterior fasciculus of left bundle branch

  Left anterior descending artery supply blood to anterior wall of left ventricle, anterior 2/3rd interventricular septum, bundle of his, right bundle branch and left anterior fasciculus of left bundle branch

- The right coronary artery divides into marginal arteries, nodal arteries, and posterior interventricular branch.

  Right coronary artery supply blood to right atrium, right ventricles and inferior part of left ventricle

  Posterior interventricular artery supply blood to posterior 1/3rd of interventricular septum

Various anastomoses and collaterals are formed between branches of the left and right coronary artery. No symptoms of Ischemic Heart Disease (IHD) are noticeable until more than 70% of coronary artery lumen is occluded.

The risk of myocardial infarction increases when more than 90% of the arterial lumen is occluded.

- In 90% population, branches of right coronary artery supplies SA and AV node (right dominant heart). Posterior descending artery arises from the right coronary artery.

- In 10% population, branches of left coronary artery supplies SA and AV node (left dominant heart). Posterior descending artery arises from left coronary artery.

Cardiac veins will collect blood from the capillaries of the myocardium and will drain into the coronary sinus. Coronary sinus will drain this deoxygenated blood back to the right atrium.

Blood supply to the heart

- The heart receives blood supply during diastole because the aortic valve closes and opens the pathway for blood to enter coronary vessels.

- The increase in heart rate (tachycardia) will have a shorter diastolic period and thus decreased filling time or decrease in cardiac output.

Coronary artery occlusion in myocardial infarction

- Left anterior descending artery is most commonly occluded cardiac artery (50% cases of MI) followed by the right coronary artery in 30% cases and left circumflex artery in 20% cases.

Innervation of the heart

- The phrenic nerve carries pain fibers from the pericardium.

- Sympathetic stimulation increases heart rate. Anginal pain signals travel by sympathetic fibers to spinal cord segment T1-T5.

- Parasympathetic stimulation decreases heart rate. Sensory nerve fibers that carry afferent limb of cardiac reflex travels via the vagus nerve.

CONCEPTS OF PRELOAD, EJECTION FRACTION AND CARDIAC OUTPUT

PRELOAD

- Preload is the load on ventricular muscle at the end of diastole. It is determined mainly by the left ventricular end diastolic volume and left ventricular end diastolic pressure, in other words - by venous return.

- The increase in preload will cause an increase in contractility, which subsequently lead to a rise in stroke volume and ejection fraction.

- The increase in pulmonary capillary wedge pressure is evidence of increased preload. In mitral stenosis or mitral valve prolapse, it is not a good index of left ventricular preload because of backward congestion leading to pulmonary edema.

- Chronic increase in preload can lead to dilated cardiomyopathy.

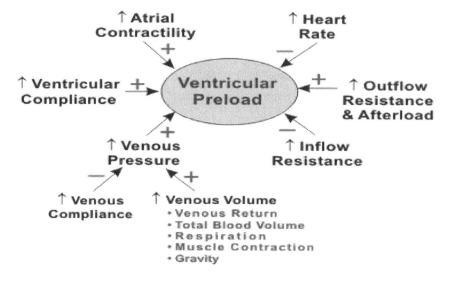

Figure 3.1: effects on the ventricular preload

STROKE VOLUME

- Stroke volume is the amount of blood that heart pumps out with each beat. It is directly proportional to contractility of the heart and inversely proportional to afterload.

- Stroke volume is calculated as -

  SV = EDV (End Diastolic Volume) – ESV (End Systolic Volume).

EJECTION FRACTION

- Ejection fraction Is the portion of blood that heart pumps out **during one contraction**, which is usually 60-70% in the healthy normal adult.

- Ejection fraction is calculated as:

  Ejection Fraction = stroke volume/end diastolic volume

  Now, SV = EDV – ESV, and therefore, **EF** = EDV – ESV/EDV

- For example; If the SV is 70 ml and EDV is 120 ml in 70kg man. Therefore, ejection fraction is 60% in this individual

CARDIAC OUTPUT

- Cardiac output is the amount of blood that heart pumps out during 1 minute.

- Cardiac output is calculated as **CO =** heart rate * stroke volume.

  For example; If the heart rate is 72/min, and stroke volume is 70 ml. Therefore cardiac output in 1 minute = 5000ml or 5 L/min.

- According to the Fick's principle, **CO =** rate of oxygen consumption / arterial oxygen content – venous oxygen content.

AFTERLOAD

- Afterload is the pressure against which heart will work. It is determined by peripheral arterial resistance.

- Chronic increase in afterload (e.g. hypertension, increasing age) will lead to left ventricular hypertrophy. Peripheral resistance is calculated as -

  Blood flow = pressure/resistance (Q=P/R), therefore **R** = P/Q

  Resistance is inversely proportional to the 4th power of the radius of the vessel.

  If the resistance will increase, then the blood flow will decrease and the heart will have to do more work to pump out blood against more resistance.

  Chronically it will lead to systolic dysfunction (impaired contractility) and diastolic dysfunction (impaired ventricular relaxation).

- Hypotension occurs when afterload is decreased (e.g. septic shock)

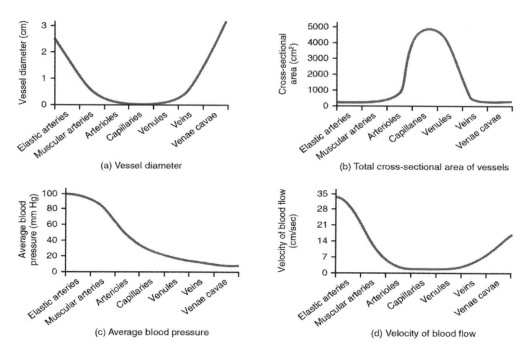

Figure 3.2: graphical representation of the vascular diameter, cross-sectional area, blood pressure and velocity of blood flow*

- The total cross-sectional area of capillaries is more than aorta or vena cava.

- The aorta has the largest diameter but has smallest total cross-sectional area

Total flow is calculated as:

- **Flow =** pressure/resistance or Q = P/R
- **Flow =** cross sectional area * velocity of flow or Q = A*V or V = Q/A

- Based on this equation, we can say that the velocity of flow decreases when total cross-sectional area increases and vice versa.

  Therefore, capillary will have the least velocity of blood flow when compared to aorta and vena cava because capillaries have largest cross-sectional area.

- Another formula to calculate flow across pulmonary vessels is -

  Q = oxygen consumption / Po2 pulmonary vein – Po2 pulmonary artery

  = 250 ml/min / 0.20ml/min – 0.15 ml/min = 5000 ml/min.

Autoregulation mechanism dominates over extrinsic mechanism (neuronal and hormonal influences). Because the gastrointestinal system does not have dominant autoregulation system, their vessels will constrict under SNS activity, and therefore, blood flow decreases to the gastrointestinal system during exercise.

1) Coronary circulation: auto-regulated by endogenous *adenosine and nitric oxide*. When the heart is under stress, more ATP will be used up, and adenosine will form as a byproduct. Adenosine dilates coronary vessels and provides sufficient blood flow to the heart to meet its energy requirements.

2) Cerebral circulation: brain maintains its circulation mainly by arterial carbon dioxide level ($PaCO_2$). During exercise, cerebral circulation is unchanged because exercise will increase the level of venous blood carbon dioxide level, which subsequently undergoes pulmonary oxygenation before reaching to the brain.

3) Skeletal muscle (during exercise only): skeletal muscle during exercise regulate its blood flow with the help of myogenic stretch receptors (pressure related) and vasodilator metabolites like lactate. In resting muscle, flow is controlled mainly by the sympathetic nervous system (alpha-1 and beta-2 receptors).

4) Renal blood flow: blood flow to the kidney is also commonly considered as autoregulation even though neuronal and hormonal influences partially control it. During hypertension, renal afferents will constrict and maintains its blood flow to the kidney. Chronically, it will lead to hypertensive nephropathy.

5) Cutaneous blood flow: heat causes vasodilation and cold temperature causes vasoconstriction. During fever and exercise, there is an increase in heat loss which causes flushing due to vasodilation.

ORGAN SYSTEM	CHANGE IN BLOOD FLOW DURING EXERCISE
Coronary	Increases
Pulmonary	Increases
Cerebral	No change
Renal	Decrease
Gastrointestinal	Decrease
Exercising muscle	Increases
Cutaneous	Increases

Table 3.1: changes in blood flow to various organ systems during exercise

LAMINAR FLOW and TURBULENT FLOW

Normally, we have laminar blood flow throughout the body except the flow in the heart and conducting airways of respiratory tree (due to excessive vessel branching).

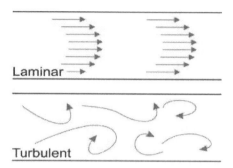

Figure 3.3: laminar flow and turbulent flow

The layer with the highest velocity is in the center of the vessels.

Heavier particles like unactivated neutrophils and platelets flow in the center of the vessel while lighter particles flow at the periphery. This is because the center of flow will have the least resistance while the periphery will have maximum resistance.

Activation of cells like neutrophils or platelets due to endothelial injury or inflammatory process will pull them toward the periphery and the 1st step of inflammation will occur.

Turbulent flow is a non-layered flow that creates murmur. This can be heard as bruits in narrowed vessels (e.g. atherosclerosis of renal artery). The high velocity of blood flow can also create turbulent flow and can cause bruits (e.g. anemia).

- Reynold's number can calculate the type of flow;

  Reynold's number = diameter * velocity * density / viscosity

- According to this formula, diameter, velocity, and density of blood are directly proportional to turbulent flow and viscosity is inversely proportional to turbulent flow. You do not need to remember specific numbers for the exam.

- The increase in blood viscosity is seen in polycythemia, lung diseases (hypoxia-induced erythropoietin production from the kidney), multiple myeloma and hereditary spherocytosis.

- The decrease in blood viscosity is seen in anemia.

- Resistance is directly proportional to the viscosity of blood and length of the vessel, and it is inversely proportional to the 4th power of the radius.

  R α viscosity * length /radius

  It means when the radius of artery decreases by ½ (50%), resistance will increase by 16 times (½* ½ * ½ * ½) and when the radius of artery increases by ½ (50%), resistance will decrease by 16 times.

- The increase in total peripheral resistance is the leading cause of primary hypertension worldwide. This accounts for 95% of hypertensive cases (4% is due to renal artery stenosis and 1% due to all other secondary causes of high blood pressure).

- This is the reason, why many cardiac or antihypertensive pharmacological therapy is aimed to decrease total peripheral resistance.

- Arterioles offer maximum resistance, and thus the steepest decrease in blood pressure will occur at this point.

$$Series: \quad \overset{R_1}{\text{—}\wedge\wedge\wedge} \overset{R_2}{\text{—}\wedge\wedge\wedge} \overset{R_3}{\text{—}\wedge\wedge\wedge\text{—}} = \overset{R_{eq}=R_1+R_2+R_3}{\text{—}\wedge\wedge\wedge\text{—}}$$

$$Parallel: \quad \begin{array}{c} R_1 \\ R_2 \\ R_3 \end{array} = \overset{R_{eq}=(1/R_1+1/R_2+1/R_3)^{-1}}{\text{—}\wedge\wedge\wedge\text{—}}$$

RESISTANCE IN SERIES CIRCUIT

- It is calculated as the sum of all resistance: R1+R2+R3 = R (maximum).

- An example of series connection is aorta-intestinal vessels-liver-inferior vena cava. The total resistance will be higher than individual resistance.

  When R2 is constricted, the pressure at R1 increases and the pressure at R3 decreases. Clinically speaking, blood pressure distal to narrowed point will be low (for example: In coarctation of aorta in adults, blood pressure will be higher in upper extremities when compared to lower extremities)

- This concept can also be applied in pulmonary edema due to congestive heart failure. When left heart fails to pump out blood (due to aortic stenosis, chronic hypertension or myocardial infarction), hydrostatic pressure will increase in pulmonary circulation and, extravasation of transudate (protein-free fluid) occurs in lung interstitium, which will lead to one of the classic finding of the left heart failure - dyspnea.

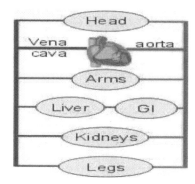

Figure 3.4: series connections (aorta-GI-liver-vena cava-heart-aorta) and parallel connections (head-arms-GI or liver-kidney-legs)

RESISTANCE IN PARALLEL CIRCUIT

- Resistance in a parallel circuit is calculated as the sum of the inverse of resistance: $1/R1 + 1/R2 + 1/R3 = 1/R$ (minimum).

- An example of parallel connection is pancreas-spleen-kidney-skin/bone.

- Total resistance will be lower than individual resistance.

- This concept can be applied in pregnancy where the fetus is connected to the parallel circuit. Total peripheral resistance will decrease, which will indirectly increase cardiac output in pregnant. Blood pressure will not increase unless gestational hypertension develops.

- This concept can also be applied in organ transplantation. When a donor donates his kidney, total peripheral resistance increases because the parallel circuit is removed. This will indirectly decrease cardiac output.

- Coronary arteries have the greatest resistance while pulmonary circulation has the least resistance.

- The primary factor that determines systolic blood pressure is stroke volume.

  The increase in preload or increase in contractility will increase stroke volume, which will increase systolic blood pressure.

  Decrease in compliance of vessels (age-related arteriosclerosis) also increases systolic blood pressure (isolated systolic hypertension).

 The primary factor determining diastolic blood pressure is total peripheral resistance.

THUNDERNOTE: Effect of Position Change on Blood Pressure

- We measure lower extremity blood pressure by asking the patient to lay down on their stomach because, in standing position, pressure in lower extremities will be very high due to the effect of gravity (around 180mmHg) and the pressure above the heart will be less (lower than 120mmHg).

- When pressure decreases above the heart in an upright position, carotid sinus reflex will immediately fire, increasing total peripheral resistance and heart rate to maintain enough perfusion to the brain. This is the reason standing person will have a rapid heart rate or contraction as compared to a person laying down.

SYSTEMIC CIRCULATION (mmHg)		PULMONARY CIRCULATION (mmHg)	
Left ventricle	120/0	Right ventricle	25/0
Aorta	120/80	Pulmonary artery	25/8
Mean arterial pressure	93	Mean pulmonary artery pressure	15
Renal glomerular	50	Pulmonary capillary	7-10
Peripheral veins	15	Pulmonary veins	5
Right atrium (central venous pressure)	0-5	Left atrium	5-10
Pressure gradient	93-0 = 93	Pressure gradient	15-5 = 10

Table 3.2: pressure in the systemic and pulmonary circulation

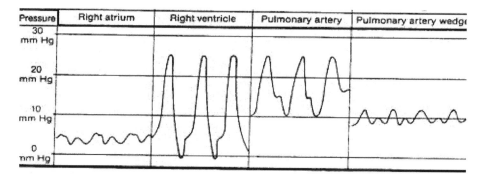

Figure 3.5: pulmonary pressure curve by flow directed catheter

MEAN ARTERIAL PRESSURE

- Mean arterial pressure is the average arterial pressure during the cardiac cycle.

- It is calculated as: **MAP** = cardiac output * total peripheral resistance.

  MAP = 2/3rd diastolic pressure + 1/3rd systolic pressure.

  If an individual has blood pressure of 120/80 mmHg,

  MAP = 2/3rd (80) + 1/3rd (120) = **92 mmHg**

- During static and high-intensity exercise like weight lifting, a physical compression of blood vessels raises total peripheral resistance. The increase in total peripheral resistance will increase the blood pressure.

- Dynamic and aerobic exercises will not significantly affect mean blood pressure (minor isolated systolic rise in blood pressure can be seen) because the decrease in total peripheral resistance (due to dilation of arterioles in exercising muscle) is accompanied by an equivalent increase in cardiac output.

- Mean arterial pressure is not equal to mean systemic pressure.

MEAN SYSTEMIC PRESSURE

- Mean systemic pressure is the average pressure that exists in the vascular system if the cardiac output stops and the pressure within the vascular system redistributes.

- It is an indicator of how full the circulatory system is.

- Value of mean systemic pressure is nearly equal to right atrial pressure - 3-8mmHg

- Right atrial pressure is also called as central venous pressure.

- Mean systemic pressure depends on the total compliance of the arterial, venous beds and the total blood volume within them.

THUNDERNOTE: HYPERTHYROIDISM

Few pathologies that increase sympathetic tone are:

- Hyperthyroidism

- Pheochromocytoma

- Obstructive sleep apnea

The high sympathetic tone will cause constriction of arterioles. This will increase systolic blood pressure more than diastolic pressure.

GRAVES DISEASE

- Classic symptoms are those of hyperthyroidism which includes palpitation, anxiety, hand tremors, weight loss, pretibial myxedema and exophthalmos (fibroblasts in the orbital tissues may express the TSH receptor which causes accumulation of glycosaminoglycan behind the eyeball).

- Continuous stimulation of TSH receptors by anti-thyroglobulin antibodies will release a high amount of T4 and T3 in circulation. The high level of thyroid hormones will decrease TRH and TSH production by negative feedback on the hypothalamus.

- Ventricular fibrillation is the most common cause of death in Grave's disease.

- The patient is treated with propranolol and methimazole or propylthiouracil.

SUBACUTE THYROIDITIS

- De quervain's subacute thyroiditis is a self-limiting disease that usually occurs after a viral infection. It can manifest clinically with symptoms of hyperthyroidism and hypothyroidism.

- Hyperthyroidism occurs due to the destruction of thyroid cells, which releases thyroid hormone into the bloodstream. Once cells get destroyed, the phase of hypothyroidism begins.

- The thyroid gland is **tender** and painful on palpation.

- On lab findings, ESR is classically elevated.

- The patient is treated symptomatically with beta-blockers and NSAIDs. Propylthiouracil and methimazole are not indicated.

- **Compliance** means the ability of the vessel to get stretch (dilate). If the vessel is easily stretched, it is considered to be highly compliant.

  Compliance is inversely related to elasticity.

- **Elasticity** is the tendency to rebound back to original size from a stretch.

  A vessel with high elasticity will have low compliance.

Factors affecting compliance:

- **Endothelial dysfunction** reduces compliance due to increase in arterial stiffness.

  This phenomenon is seen in hypertensive, diabetes, and smokers. Atherosclerosis will further aggravate this stiffness.

  Pulse contour analysis is a non-invasive method that allows easy measurement of arterial elasticity to identify patients at risk for cardiovascular events.

- **Age:** Newborn will have higher compliant vessels compared to 50-year-old man.

  With the increase in age, compliance will decrease, and elasticity will increase. The less compliant artery will increase the total peripheral resistance that sometimes causes a pseudo-increase in blood pressure during blood pressure measurement in an elderly patient.

- Fish oil alters vascular reactivity and favorably influences arterial wall characteristics in patients with non-insulin dependent diabetes mellitus.

- Venous compliance is approximately 25 times larger than arterial compliance and contains nearly 70% of systemic blood volume. Arteries are high-pressure vessels and are very stiff because of the high muscular layer and therefore, arteries do not represent a significant blood reservoir. The aorta is most compliant in the arterial system.

- Compliance is calculated using the following equation, where ΔV is the change in volume, and ΔP is the change in pressure; $C = \Delta V/ \Delta P$

- Pulse pressure will increase while going distally from the aorta (because compliance decreases). The pedal artery will have higher pulse pressure than femoral artery and femoral artery will have higher pulse pressure than the aorta.

PULSE PRESSURE

- Pulse pressure is the difference between systolic pressure and diastolic pressure.

- It is calculated as:

  PP = systolic pressure – diastolic pressure.

Other factors that can widen pulse pressure are:

- Increase in stroke volume (during exercise, systolic pressure increases more than diastolic pressure)

- Decrease in vessel compliance (as we grow older, compliance decreases. Therefore older people have higher pulse pressure compared to younger ones).

- The compliant artery will have a small pulse pressure and stiffened artery will have significant pulse pressure.

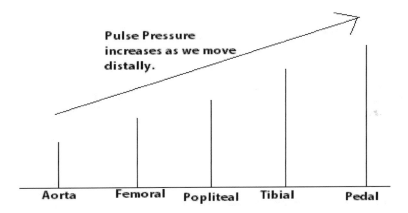

Figure 3.6: pulse pressure change*

- As we go distally from the heart, pulse pressure increases because diastolic blood pressure and compliance of vessel decreases.

- This concept is applicable to arteries only because pulse pressure does not take into consideration of venous system.

- If you are presented with any vein in multiple choices on an exam, do not select that answer because if calculated, veins will always have lower pulse pressure compared to arteries.

THUNDERNOTE: PHYSIOLOGICAL CHANGES IN PREGNANCY

- During the pregnancy plasma volume increases by 50%, which increases preload. The maximum increase in plasma volume occurs during first two trimesters of gestation. The rise in preload will increase contractility of the heart and stroke volume increases by 30%.

- Total peripheral resistance decreases due to the parallel connection of fetus. This will increase the heart rate by about 20%.

- The rise in heart rate and stroke volume will cause an increase in cardiac output by approximately 50% (CO = HR * SV). This massive increase in cardiac output will cause systolic ejection murmur along the left sternal border and it is perfectly normal during pregnancy. Do not confuse this murmur with hypertrophic obstructive cardiomyopathy or aortic stenosis.

- The **inferior vena cava syndrome** is a positional hypotension that occurs due to the compression of inferior vena cava by the uterus when a pregnant woman lies in the supine position. This compression decreases venous return and also decreases cardiac output. Management of this syndrome is to ask a pregnant woman to lie on her left lateral position. However, diastolic murmurs are never normal, and they must be investigated further.

- Central venous pressure is unchanged in pregnancy but femoral venous pressure increases by 2-3 times by the end of 2nd trimester. This increase in femoral venous pressure will cause **varicose veins or hemorrhoids** (very common) in a pregnant woman. This pathology resolves after the delivery.

- Typically, blood pressure decreases during pregnancy by 10-20 mmHg. It is never elevated physiologically in pregnancy. Both systolic and diastolic blood pressure starts falling by the end of the first trimester of pregnancy. Lowest blood pressure in the pregnancy is at around 24th week. After 24 weeks, blood pressure increases again till delivery. Even though blood pressure increases, it does not go above the pre-pregnancy measurements.

  Gestational hypertension, pre-eclampsia, and eclampsia are three conditions where blood pressure pathologically increases to very high level. Eclampsia is defined as preeclampsia + seizures.

- Other things that are considered normal for a pregnant woman is an increase in ESR, clotting factors (increased risk of deep venous thrombosis), WBC count, RBC mass and decrease in hematocrit (dilutional effect due to high plasma volume).

- The stroke volume of the heart increases in response to the rise in volume of blood filling the heart (end diastolic volume) when all other factors remain constant.

- The increased volume of blood (preload) stretches the ventricular wall, causing the cardiac muscle to contract more forcefully. The stroke volume may also increase as a result of greater contractility of the cardiac muscle during exercise, independent of the end-diastolic volume.

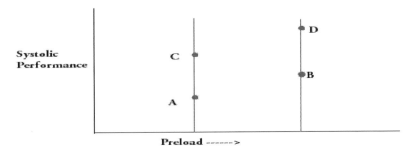

Figure 3.7: performance change with increase in preload and contractility*

Suppose point A is normal functioning heart,

- When preload is increased (e.g. on laying down), point A will move to point B. This increase in performance is entirely due to preload.

- In response to increasing preload, a healthy heart will increase its contractility and shift point B to D. Therefore, increase in performance from point A to point D is combined effect of preload and contractility (e.g. exercise).

- If contractility is independently increased (e.g. digoxin, dobutamine), it would shift the heart performance from point A to point C. Thus, point A to C is entirely due to increasing in contractility.

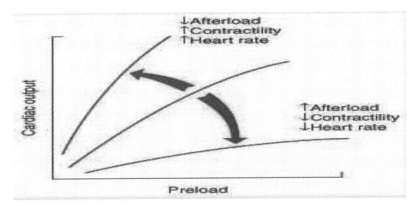

Figure 3.8: effects of preload, afterload, contractility and heart rate on cardiac output*

- When line shifts to left (upward), contractility increases and when line shift to right (downward) contractility decreases.

  Various positive inotropic drugs like digoxin, catecholamine and exercise will cause an increase in contractility.

  Negative inotropic drugs (beta-blockers, calcium channel blockers), dilated cardiomyopathy and heart failure will cause a decrease in contractility.

PHYSIOLOGICAL PARAMETERS AND DRUGS

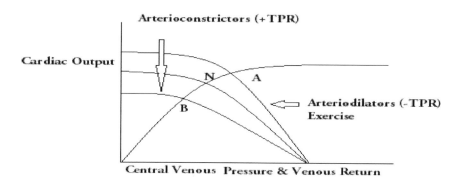

Figure 3.9: effect of vasoconstrictors and vasodilators on the central venous pressure and venous return*

This concept is what we discussed earlier, but the boards (especially step 1) will test you with all these different graphs, and you should be prepared for all.

- **Point N** is the normal operating point of the heart on the standard line.

- **Point A:** when the peripheral resistance is decreased (hydralazine, exercise), cardiac output will increase. This will shift the line above the standard line. Venous return will also increase due to high cardiac output (point N to A)

  There is not net gain or loss of volume, therefore central venous pressure (right atrial pressure) remains constant (1 point on the x-axis).

- **Point B:** when the peripheral resistance is increased (norepinephrine or phenylephrine), cardiac output will decrease. This will shift the line below the standard line. Venous return will also fall due to low cardiac output (point N to B)

  There is no net gain or loss of volume, therefore central venous pressure remains constant (1 point on the x-axis).

PHYSIOLOGICAL PARAMETERS AND CHANGE IN PLASMA VOLUME

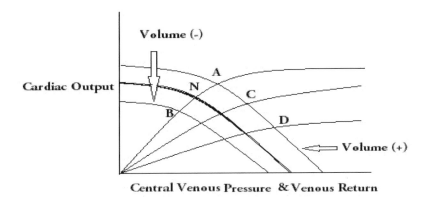

Figure 3.10: effect of change in volume on the central venous pressure and venous return*

- **Point A:** whenever blood volume increases (saline/plasma infusion), the cardiac output will increase (remember muscle mechanics; when muscles are stretched within physiological limit, the contractility of muscle increases). This will increase venous return (point N to A).

  There is gain of volume, therefore central venous pressure will also increase (right shift of regular line on x-axis)

- **Point B:** whenever blood volume decreases (severe bleeding), the cardiac output will decrease. This will decrease venous return (point N to B)

  There is loss of volume, therefore central venous pressure will also drop (left shift of regular line on x-axis)

- **Point D:** this point represents decompensated heart failure (heart is stretched beyond the physiological limit and, therefore, failure to achieve maximum contraction even when preload is high).

  Central venous pressure is tremendously increased. The mechanism behind this is not due to high venous return, but because of backward failure and venous congestion.

- **Point C:** this point represents compensated heart failure (digoxin therapy will cause increase in cardiac output by increasing contractility of heart)

  Even with best therapy, we cannot achieve a cardiac output, as like healthy heart and so this point will always remain below the standard point.

THUNDERNOTE: PHYSIOLOGICAL PARAMETERS AND ATRIOVENOUS FISTULA

In acute AV fistula; there will be 1 junction point on x-axis

In chronic AV fistula; new point will shift to the right on x-axis

- Acutely, AV fistula causes a decrease in peripheral resistance, which increases cardiac output and venous return. However, venous return curve does not immediately shift along the x-axis.

- Over the period of time, the sympathetic activity and kidney will begin to compensate by increasing cardiac contractility, vascular tone, and circulating blood volume. These changes will increase the cardiac function curve and mean systemic pressure, which causes an increase in venous return (right shift on the x-axis).

- AV fistula can cause high-output cardiac failure

ACTION POTENTIAL

Special types of voltage-gated ion channels are embedded in a cell's plasma membrane which generates an action potential. They handle the generation of electrical impulses in the heart.

Fast response fibers (atrial and ventricular myocardium, His-purkinje system)

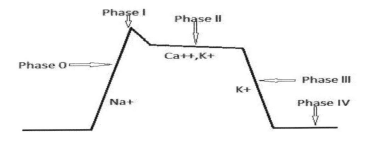

Figure 3.11: cardiac action potentials in fast response fibers

Resting membrane potential is the voltage difference between the inside of the membrane and outside of the membrane.

Intracellular environment of the cell has negative RMP (-90mV). When cell is appropriately stimulated, positive charges such as sodium and calcium will go into the cell and increase the RMP. When the membrane potential will reach to its threshold (-70mV), the voltage gated sodium channels opens and rapid influx of sodium (positive ions) occurs which will increase the membrane potential to +10mV. This event is called depolarization **(phase 0).**

Class I antiarrhythmic like procainamide blocks phase 0 in fast response fibers.

Phase 1 is called overshoot and clinically insignificant. Sodium channels are inactivated during this phase. Overshoot develops because of slow potassium current going out of the cell and chlorine coming into the cell. No drugs act on this phase.

After the cell is depolarized, depolarized-sensitive calcium and potassium channel starts opening. The level of intracellular potassium (positive charge ion) is higher than extracellular potassium and the level of extracellular calcium (positive charge ion) is higher than intracellular calcium. For a brief duration, potassium is going out and calcium is coming in the cell and keep balance in the electromagnetic voltage across the cell membrane **(phase 2).**

As the time passes, delayed-rectified potassium channel opens and heavy efflux of potassium occur from the intracellular to extracellular environment and RMP return back to -90mV (due to concentration dependent efflux of positive ions). This phenomenon is called repolarization **(phase 3).**

After the repolarization phase, Na+/K+ ATPase pump will send 2 sodium ions out of the cell in exchange for 3 potassium ions. This will help to replete ion concentration inside and outside the cell **(phase 4).**

This whole process of depolarization and repolarization is called as action potential. When the cell is undergoing depolarization, some of these sodium will go to the next cell via gap junction and resting membrane potassium reaches threshold of adjacent cell and leading to its depolarization and repolarization. This cell will stimulate another adjacent cell and the action potential pass over the entire myocardium.

Action potential in slow response fibers (SA and AV nodes)

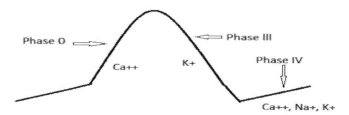

Figure 3.12: cardiac action potentials in slow response fibers

- **Phase 0 (depolarization phase):** this phase depends on the calcium channels and not on the sodium channels. With each depolarization, SA node will send signals to contract the heart. Class IV antiarrhythmic like verapamil and diltiazem will slow down this phase.

- **Phase I & II is not present** in SA and AV node

- **Phase III** (repolarization phase): this phase mainly depends on potassium going out of the cell.

- **Phase IV (raising slope):** this phase is also referred to as pacemaker current. It is mainly due to the inward sodium-calcium currents and outward potassium currents. Parasympathetic nervous system, beta-blockers, and calcium channel blockers act on this phase and decrease the heart rate.

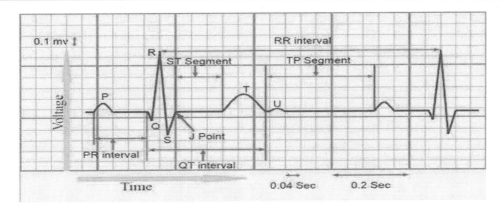

Figure 3.13: normal ECG

- **P-wave** is generated due to atrial depolarization. It indicates sinus rhythm.

- **PR interval** is due to the conduction delay through AV node (normally < 200 msec). It gets prolonged in AV blocks.

PR prolonged in AV block

- **QRS complex** is due to the ventricular depolarization (normally < 120 msec).

- **QT interval** is the total time period of mechanical contraction of ventricles

- **T wave** is generated due to ventricular repolarization. QRS complex masks atrial repolarization.

- **U wave** is small upstroke after T wave that can be seen in hypokalemia.

- SA node determines the heart activity. The normal rate of firing SA node is 80-100/min, AV node is 40-60/min, and Bundle of His/Purkinje is 20-40/min. Idioventricular rhythm is diagnosed when there is no p wave present, and ventricles are contracting under AV nodal rhythm.

- The distance between 2 R-R waves is used to determine the heart rate. It is not helpful if the rhythm is irregular.

  If distance between R-R wave of adjacent complex is 1 big box, heart rate is 300 beats/min, 2 boxes = 150 beats/min, 3 boxes = 100 beats/min, 4 boxes = 75 beats/min, 5 boxes = 60 beats/min, 6 boxes = 50 beats/min.

- Another method for determining the rate of irregular rhythms is to multiply the number of QRS complex in rhythm strip II (a bottom strip that runs through entire ECG paper) with 6.

SYMPATHETIC NERVOUS SYSTEM	
Receptors	**Characteristics**
α1 (Gq-coupled)	• Receptors are predominantly present on arteriole system. • Stimulation will constrict arterioles, which will increase both systolic and diastolic blood pressure.
β1 (Gs-coupled)	• Receptors are predominantly present all over the heart. • Stimulation will increase the heart rate (positive chronotropic), the conduction velocity of action potentials (positive dromotropic), and contractility (positive inotropic).
α2 (Gi-coupled)	• Stimulation will decrease the release and synthesis of norepinephrine (main SNS neurotransmitter). • Potential side effects of α2 agonist drugs are platelet aggregation and decrease in insulin release.
β 2 (Gs-coupled)	• The β2 action is to dilate vessels (decreases diastolic blood pressure). • They are mainly influenced by epinephrine (2nd main neurotransmitter of SNS – synthesized by adrenal medulla). • SNS fibers do not innervate β2 receptors, therefore, epinephrine acts directly on the receptors.
PARASYMPATHETIC NERVOUS SYSTEM	
M2 (Gi-coupled)	• Muscarinic type 2 receptors are located only in the atrium. • Stimulation of M2 receptors will decrease the heart rate (negative chronotropic) and conduction velocity (negative dromotropic). They do not have any effects on contractility.

(handwritten annotation: THR + Chronotropic)

Table 3.3: effect of adrenergic and cholinergic receptors on the cardiovascular system

- The dominant effect of SNS is mediated by α1 and β1 receptors. α2 and β2 action will become dominant when any drug will block α1 and β1 receptors.

- α1 decreases renin release while β1 increases renin release.

- There are many other systemic effects of these receptors. Don't forget about them while combining medications.

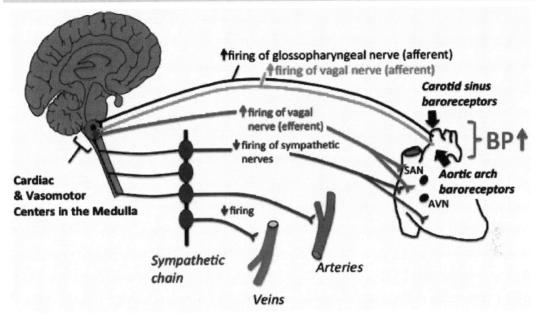

Figure 3.14: baroreceptor reflexes*

- Baroreceptors are located in the carotid sinus and aortic arch. The afferent nerve fibers from carotid sinus are carried by the glossopharyngeal nerve (cranial nerve IX) and the afferent nerve fibers from carotid sinus are carried by the vagus nerve (cranial nerve X). These afferent fibers end in the nucleus of tractus solitaries in the medulla. Nucleus of tractus solitaries thereafter sends:

  1) Inhibitory fibers to sympathetic preganglionic nucleus located in the lateral horn of spinal nucleus.

  2) Excitatory fibers to dorsal nucleus of vagus nerve (regulates parasympathetic response)

  (many interconnections of both excitatory and inhibitory neurons exist. Final net effect is inhibitory)

- When the blood pressure increases, the stretch will be felt by these baroreceptors, and they will fire more signals. The rise in baroreceptor firing will cause an increase in nucleus solitarius firing. This will increase the firing of inhibitory-excitatory neurons causing the decrease in sympathetic effect and increase in parasympathetic effect. This will decrease the heart rate and total peripheral resistance.

- The reverse phenomenon occurs when blood pressure falls. These reflexes are very rapid. In the patient with sudden onset of supraventricular tachycardia, doing carotid massage and valsalva maneuver will immediately increase baroreceptor firings and will alleviate SVTs.

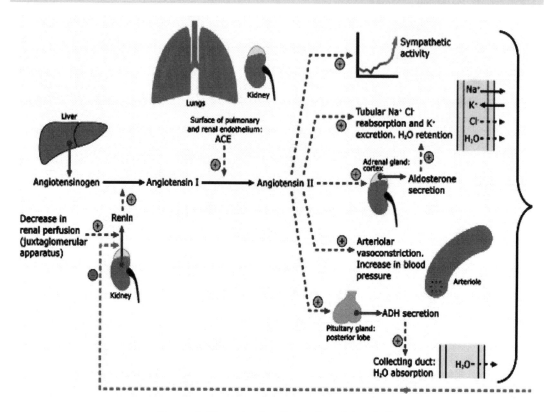

Figure 3.15: systemic effects of angiotensin II

The RAAS is a hormone system that regulates blood pressure and water (fluid) balance.

- When blood volume is low, juxtaglomerular cells in the kidney will secrete renin directly into circulation.

- Plasma renin will convert angiotensinogen (released by the liver) to angiotensin I. Angiotensin I will be subsequently converted to angiotensin II by the enzyme angiotensin-converting enzyme (target for ACE-inhibitors) in the lungs.

Effects of Angiotensin II

- Angiotensin II activates sympathetic nervous system activity that causes blood vessels to constrict, increasing blood pressure.

- Angiotensin II also stimulates secretion of hormone aldosterone from the adrenal cortex. Aldosterone causes the tubules of kidneys to increase the reabsorption of sodium and water into the blood in exchange for potassium and acid. This will increase the plasma volume and raises the blood pressure.

- Angiotensin II also acts on the posterior pituitary, which will increase antidiuretic hormone secretion (ADH). ADH is a hormone that acts on distal collecting tubules and facilitates water absorption independent of sodium. If the renin-angiotensin-aldosterone system is abnormally active, blood pressure will be high. There are many drugs that interrupt different steps in this system to lower blood pressure. These drugs are one of the main ways to control high blood pressure, heart failure, kidney failure, and harmful effects of diabetes.

ATRIAL NATRIURETIC PEPTIDE and BRAIN NATRIURETIC PEPTIDE

- Increase in a stretch of right atrium and ventricle will release ANP (Atrial Natriuretic Peptides) and BNP (Brain Natriuretic Peptide) respectively. Both of them play a minor role in maintaining blood pressure by diuresis and vasodilation.

- Unlike RAS system, this diuretic process is not rapid or powerful. Determining BNP level have only one clinical significance; to detect the dilation of ventricles.

- Due to this reason, **nesiritide** (recombinant BNP) is never the correct answer on the board exams for first and second line drugs in heart failure. In fact, Nesiritide has not shown any decrease in mortality.

ANTIDIURETIC HORMONE

- The posterior pituitary secretes ADH. It's secretion increases when the **volume** of blood decreases.

- ADH promotes water reabsorption by regulating aquaporin channels on the luminal side of distal convoluted tubules. Mechanoreceptors and osmoreceptors that regulate ADH secretion are located on the anterior side of the hypothalamus called as area postrema.

These are some predominant mechanisms that play vital roles in regulating blood volume, osmolality, and pressure.

Note: Do not confuse these osmoreceptors with chemoreceptors. Peripheral chemoreceptors are located in the carotid and aortic bodies while central chemoreceptors are located in the ventero-lateral surface of the medulla oblongata. The role of chemoreceptors in controlling heart rate is still debated. They play a primary role in respiration.

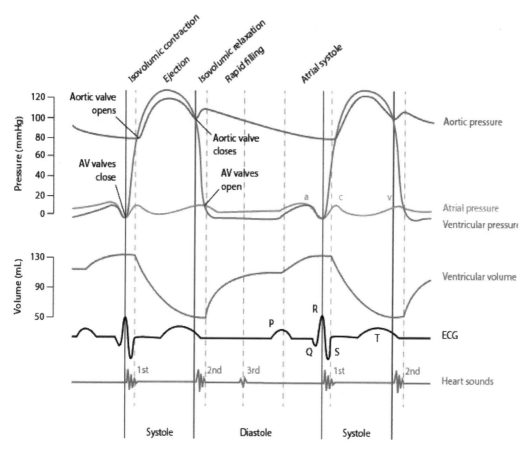

Figure 3.16: phases of cardiac cycle

5 phases of cardiac cycle are as follow:

Isovolumetric Ventricular Contraction

- Volume in the ventricles does not change during this phase.
- In response to ventricular depolarization, tension in the ventricles increases. This increase in pressure within the ventricles leads to closure of the mitral and tricuspid valves that give rise to the S1 heart sound.
- The pulmonic and aortic valves stay closed during the entire phase.
- Ventricular contraction is reflected by QRS complex on the ECG.

Ejection Phase

- The pressure during the isovolumetric ventricular contraction phase gradually increases and, when the pressure exceeds aortic and pulmonary arterial pressure (i.e. at 80 mmHg), the aortic and pulmonic valve opens and the ventricles eject blood. This phase is called as ejection phase.

Isovolumetric Relaxation

- After the ejection phase, ventricles start dilating and ventricular pressure falls below the pressure in the aorta and pulmonary artery. This will cause the closure of aortic and pulmonic valves. This period is called as isovolumetric relaxation.
- The closure of pulmonary and aortic valve will produce S2 sound.
- All valves are closed during this phase and therefore, there is no net gain or loss of volume in the ventricles.
- Atrial diastole occurs during this time, and the blood fills the atria.
- Pulmonary valves close before the aortic valves that will produce split in the 2nd heart sound that can be heard during inspiration on auscultation. Anything that delays pulmonary valve closure will increase splitting.

Rapid Ventricular Filling.

- Due to the continuous return of blood from pulmonary veins, the atrial pressure will increase, and this will cause the mitral and tricuspid valves to open.
- The rapid ventricular filling is due to the passive filling of ventricles during early diastole.
- About 70% of ventricular filling takes place during this phase.
- S3 heart sound is heard during this period due to the rapid filling of ventricles.

Atrial Systole

- After rapid filling, atrial systole will occur known as the atrial kick.

- Atrial systole (coinciding with late ventricular diastole) supplies the ventricles with remaining 30% of blood for each heartbeat and the new cycle continues.

- Atrial systole is not a major factor for ventricular filling in a younger person, but it plays a significant role in ventricular filling and cardiac output in the elderly. This is the reason some elderly patients get hypotension and shortness of breath in atrial fibrillation due to backward congestion of blood resulting in pulmonary edema.

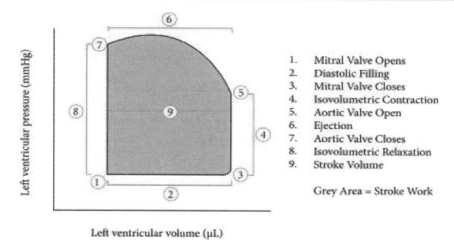

1. Mitral Valve Opens
2. Diastolic Filling
3. Mitral Valve Closes
4. Isovolumetric Contraction
5. Aortic Valve Open
6. Ejection
7. Aortic Valve Closes
8. Isovolumetric Relaxation
9. Stroke Volume

Grey Area = Stroke Work

Figure 3.17: pressure-volume loop and valvular changes

Pressure-volume loop is a graphical representation of the phases of cardiac cycle. Do not go to the exam without understanding these loops.

HYPERTENSION

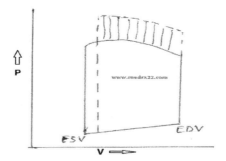

- The primary cause of hypertension in 95% of cases is high peripheral resistance. Higher force of contraction is required by the heart to pump out blood against high resistance. This will result in **high left ventricular pressure.**

- **Stroke volume will decrease** due to high peripheral resistance and, the end-systolic volume is mildly elevated.

- Initially, end diastolic volume remain unchanged due to a compensatory increase in contractility.

EXERCISE

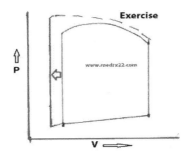

- Exercise will cause local vasodilation in exercising muscle due to the release of lactic acid and other metabolites. This will result in high cardiac output and high ejection fraction. The increase in ejection fraction will cause a mild decrease in end-systolic volume. The ventricular pressure is not significantly elevated due to peripheral vasodilation.

SYSTOLIC HEART FAILURE

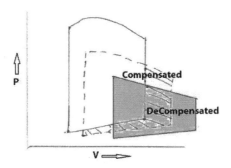

- In systolic heart failure; contractility of the heart decreases, which will result in low cardiac output. Decrease in cardiac output will cause accumulation of blood in the heart resulting in an increase in end-diastolic volume and end-systolic volume.

- Due to the decrease in efficiency of the heart, the loop moves down and right.

- Middle loop indicates partial compensation which can be seen in a patient who is on the medications that can increases cardiac output by increasing force of contraction in the heart. It is nearly impossible to achieve the functionality of heart back to the previous healthy level.

DIASTOLIC HEART FAILURE

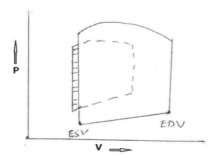

- Diastolic heart failure is a condition in which ventricles fail to dilate. Failure of dilation will not allow adequate cardiac filling during diastole. This will decrease end-diastolic volume. Due to the low preload, stroke volume decreases but ejection fraction remains normal.

- Because the heart has to pump less volume of blood, it will not be able to generate high pressure like a normal heart.

AORTIC INSUFFICIENCY (EARLY AND LATE)

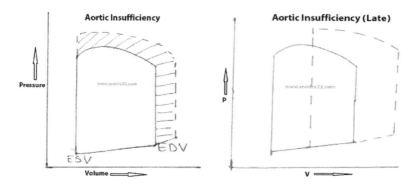

- In aortic insufficiency, blood will regurgitate back into the left ventricle. This will increase end-diastolic volume which creates a high stretch on the myocardium and this will increase the force of contraction and left ventricular pressure. This results in high ejection fraction and end-systolic volume remains unchanged.
- Over the period of time, the heart will undergo eccentric dilation due to continuous volume overload. This will result in loosening of cardiac muscle fibers and they fail to pump out the effective volume of blood. This will result in high pressure inside the ventricular cavity and increases both end systolic volume and end diastolic volume.

AORTIC STENOSIS

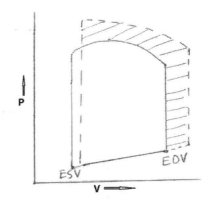

- Stenosis of the aortic valve will cause left ventricular outflow obstruction. It will generate loop similar to later stage of chronic hypertension. Ventricular outlet obstruction will not allow enough blood to go out into the systemic circulation, resulting in an increase in end-systolic volume. Even though blood returning to left ventricle will be normal, the total collection of blood in the ventricular cavity will be little higher than normal heart, i.e. high end-diastolic volume.

POSITIVE AND NEGATIVE INOTROPICS

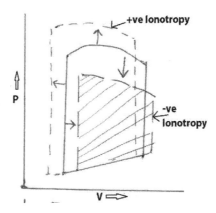

- Positive inotropes like digoxin, inamrinone, and milrinone will increase the contractility of the heart. This will result in high pressure inside the ventricles and more blood will be ejected out. Therefore, end diastolic and end systolic volume will decrease.
- Negative inotropic conditions like systolic heart failure, ventricles fail to contract and eject blood resulting in an increase in end-diastolic volume and end-systolic volume. Due to a decrease in contractility of the heart, the ventricular pressure is also decrease.

MITRAL STENOSIS

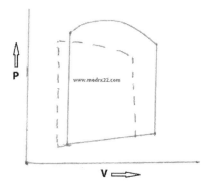

- Mitral stenosis will not allow proper filling of left ventricles resulting in a decrease in end-diastolic volume.

- Low volume of blood will not generate enough pressure during contraction. This will cause low stroke volume (due to decrease in end-diastolic volume) but the ejection fraction will be normal or slightly elevated and therefore, end systolic volume is little decreased.

MITRAL INSUFFICIENCY

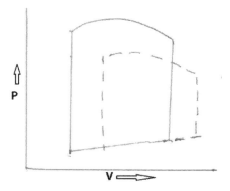

In mitral insufficiency, some amount of blood is pushed back into the left atrium during systole. Acute insufficiency (e.g. post-MI chordae tendinae rupture) will cause sudden onset of shortness of breath due to pulmonary edema but slowly developing mitral insufficiency (e.g. rheumatic valve disease) will lead to increase in end diastolic volume due to an increase in the ventricular filling (regurgitated blood along with the venous return).

Left ventricle will undergo eccentric dilation due to volume overload resulting in loop similar to systolic heart failure (low ejection fraction, high end-diastolic and end-systolic volume)

The tip of the cardiac catheter can be placed into various parts of the heart to measure the pressure within the chambers. This technique can measure various changes of pressure across the valve.

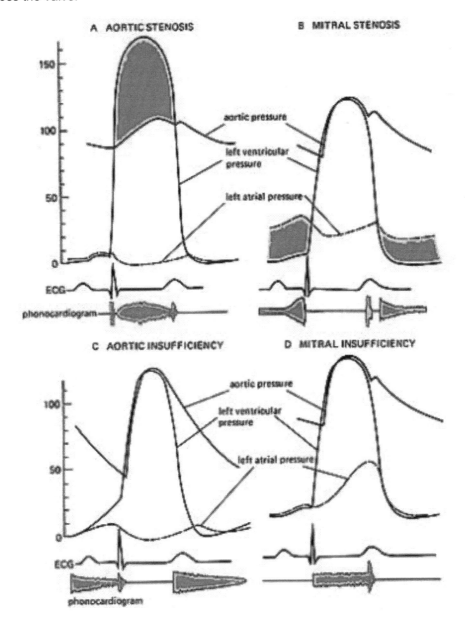

Figure 3.19: atrial and ventricular pressure change in valvular problems

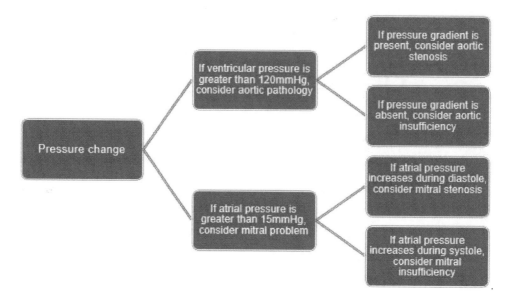

Figure 3.19.1: atrial and ventricular pressure change in valvular problems

AORTIC STENOSIS

- The ventricular pressure will be high due to the increased resistance offered by the aortic valve and the pressure inside the aortic lumen will be less because of low blood ejection. This leads to an increase in pressure gradient across the valve. The 'P' wave on ECG represents atrial contraction (diastolic phase), QRS complex represents ventricular depolarization (systolic phase) and the T wave represents ventricular repolarization, i.e. relaxation of ventricles.

MITRAL STENOSIS

- Narrow mitral valve opening impairs emptying of the left atrium during diastole resulting in an increase in left atrial pressure and volume during the diastole.

AORTIC INSUFFICIENCY

- Due to regurgitation of blood in left ventricles, the aortic pressure will decrease to a significant level during ventricular diastole. It is differentiated from aortic stenosis by the absence of pressure gradient between aortic and ventricular pressure.

MITRAL INSUFFICIENCY

- Regurgitation of blood from the left ventricles to the left atrium during systole will cause an increase in atrial pressure during systole. In mitral stenosis, atrial pressure increases during diastole while in mitral insufficiency atrial pressure increases during systole.

HEART SOUNDS

Physiologically, heart sounds are heard only on the closing of heart valves.

- **S1 heart sound** is produced due to the closure of mitral and tricuspid valves. Splitting is usually not noticeable.

- **S2 heart sound** is produced due to the closing of aortic and pulmonary valves. They are heard as a single sound during expiration, but during inspiration physiological splitting can be audible i.e. aortic valves closure (A2 component) is heard first, followed by pulmonary valve closure (P2 component). This delay occurs because right ventricular venous return increases during inspiration. Due to the increase in the volume of blood to pump into pulmonary vessels, the pulmonary valve closes with little delay as compared to the aortic valve.

S3 → filling of vent.

- **S3 heart sound** is due to rapid filling of the left ventricle. It occurs due to very compliant ventricles (eccentric cardiomyopathy). S3 sound is a normal finding in children and young adults.

- **S4 heart sound** is due to the atrial contraction against stiffened ventricles which fails to dilate adequately during the rapid filling phase. Stiff ventricles that can be seen in concentric cardiomyopathy, chronic hypertension, myocardial infarction and other conditions. S4 heart sound is almost always pathologic.

S4 → atrial kick

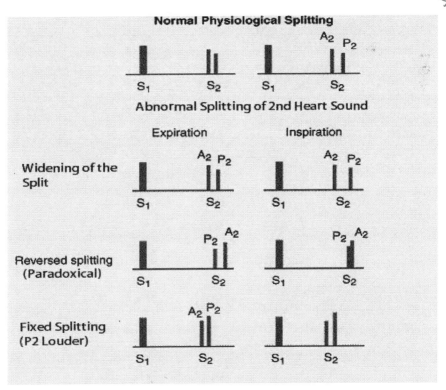

Figure 3.20: splitting of second heart sound

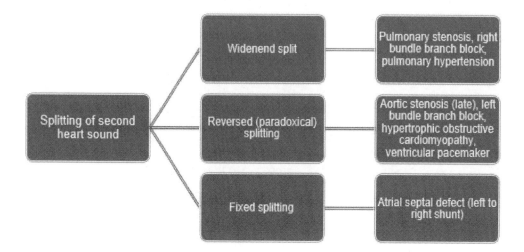

Figure 3.20.1: splitting of second heart sound

MURMURS

Murmurs are pathologic heart sounds that are produced due to turbulent blood flow in the heart that is sufficient to produce audible noise.

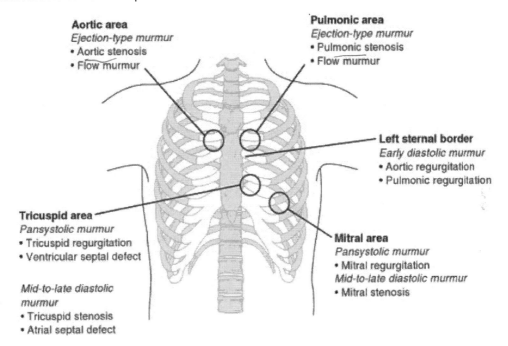

Aortic area
Ejection-type murmur
• Aortic stenosis
• Flow murmur

Pulmonic area
Ejection-type murmur
• Pulmonic stenosis
• Flow murmur

Left sternal border
Early diastolic murmur
• Aortic regurgitation
• Pulmonic regurgitation

Tricuspid area
Pansystolic murmur
• Tricuspid regurgitation
• Ventricular septal defect

Mid-to-late diastolic murmur
• Tricuspid stenosis
• Atrial septal defect

Mitral area
Pansystolic murmur
• Mitral regurgitation
Mid-to-late diastolic murmur
• Mitral stenosis

Figure 3.21: Murmurs*

GRADE	FEATURE
1	Soft, difficult to hear
2	Soft, easily heard
3	Loud, without thrill
4	Loud, with thrill
5	Loud with thrill, audible with edge of stethoscope, not audible with stethoscope just off the chest
6	Loud with thrill, audible with a stethoscope just off the chest.

Table 3.4: grading of murmurs

VALVULAR PROBLEM	PHYSICAL CHARACTERISTIC	BEST HEARD AT	OTHER FEATURES
Mitral stenosis	Late diastolic blowing murmur	Apex of heart	Opening snap, loud S1, atrial fibrillation, LAE, PH
Mitral regurgitation	Holosystolic murmur	Apex of heart, radiates to axilla	Soft S1, LAE, PH, LVH
Aortic stenosis	Harsh systolic ejection murmur	Right 2nd intercostal space, radiates to carotids	Slow pulse upstroke, s3/s4, ejection click, LVH, cardiomegaly, syncope, angina and CHF
Aortic regurgitation	Early diastolic decrescendo murmur	Left lower sternal border	Widened pulse pressure, LVH, LV dilation, S3, intensity increases with increased peripheral vascular resistance
Mitral prolapse	Mid-systolic click or late-systolic murmur, crescendo-decrescendo murmur	Usually at the apex of heart	Panic disorder

CHF - Congestive heart failure, LAE - Left atrial enlargement, LVH - Left ventricular hypertrophy, PH - Pulmonary hypertension

www.medrx-education.com

Table 3.5: valvular problems and associated findings

SYSTOLIC MURMURS

Aortic Stenosis

- Aortic stenosis produces crescendo/decrescendo systolic murmur.

- Best heard at the right upper sternal border sometimes with radiation to the carotid arteries.

- In mild aortic stenosis, the crescendo-decrescendo is early peaking whereas in severe aortic stenosis, the crescendo is late peaking, and the S2 heart sound may be obliterated.

Mitral Regurgitation

- Mitral regurgitation produces holosystolic murmur which is best heard at the apex, and may radiate to the axilla or precordium.

- The systolic click may be heard if there is associated mitral valve prolapse.

- Valsalva maneuver in mitral regurgitation associated with mitral valve prolapse will increase left ventricular preload and move the murmur onset closer to S1.

- Isometric handgrip, that increases left ventricular afterload will increase the murmur intensity.

- In acute severe mitral regurgitation, a holosystolic murmur may not be heard.

Pulmonary Stenosis

- Pulmonary stenosis produces systolic crescendo-decrescendo murmur which is best heard at the left upper sternal border.

- It can be associated with a systolic ejection click that diminishes with inspiration and sometimes radiates to the left clavicle.

Tricuspid Regurgitation

- Tricuspid regurgitation produces holosystolic murmur which is best heard at the left lower sternal border with radiation to the left upper sternal border.

- Murmur will increase with inspiration due to increased right-sided venous return during inspiration.

Hypertrophic Obstructive Cardiomyopathy

- Hypertrophic obstructive cardiomyopathy produces systolic crescendo-decrescendo murmur which is best heard at the left lower sternal border.
- Valsalva maneuver and changing position from squatting to standing will increase the intensity of the murmur.

Atrial Septal Defect/Patent Foramen Ovale

- Both conditions will cause systolic crescendo-decrescendo murmur which is best heard at the left upper sternal border due to increased volume going through the pulmonary valve. It is associated with a fixed, split S2 and a right ventricular heave.
- During the early period of the septal defect, there is a left to right shunt which maintains the oxygenation of blood. Over the long period of time, this will lead to pulmonary vessel hypertrophy and produces a pulmonary stenosis type of situation. This will increase pressure on the right side of the heart and results in a right to left shunt and poor oxygenation of blood leading to cyanosis. This phenomenon is called as Eisenmenger syndrome.

Ventricular Septal Defect

- Ventricular septal defect produces harsh holosystolic murmur which is best heard at the left lower sternal border.
- It will often have a palpable thrill, and increases with an isometric handgrip.
- Ventricular septal defect is the most common congenital heart defect.
- Eisenmenger syndrome may develop over the long period of time if left untreated.

Flow murmur (Innocent murmur)

- Flow murmur is the soft, vibratory sound at the right upper sternal border.
- It can be associated with hyperthyroidism, fever, anemia, and pregnancy.
- They are never greater than grade 2 and never heard in diastole. Reassure the patient and treat the underlying cause.

Pulmonary flow: higher pitched sound that is heard in the 2nd left parasternal space with the patient lying down.

Venous hum: heard in the neck or anterior chest. It disappears with compression of the jugular vein.

DIASTOLIC MURMUR

Aortic Regurgitation

- Aortic regurgitation produces diastolic decrescendo murmur which is best heard at the left lower sternal border or right lower sternal border (when associated with a dilated aorta).
- This may be associated with bounding carotid and peripheral pulse (Corrigan's pulse, water hammer pulse) and a widened pulse pressure.

Mitral Stenosis

- Mitral stenosis produces diastolic low-pitched decrescendo murmur which is best heard at the cardiac apex in left lateral decubitus position.
- An opening snap can be heard.
- An increase in severity will shorten the duration of time between S2 and the opening snap.
- Rheumatic heart disease is the most common cause of mitral stenosis.
- Atrial myxoma can block the outflow from left atrium and can create a condition like mitral stenosis.

Tricuspid Stenosis

- Tricuspid stenosis produces diastolic decrescendo murmur which is best heard at the left lower sternal border.
- Signs of right heart failure will be present.

Pulmonary Regurgitation

- Pulmonary regurgitation produces diastolic decrescendo murmur which is best heard at the left lower sternal border.
- A loud P2 may be heard with associated pulmonary hypertension.
- It is the least common valvular pathology.

CONTINUOUS AND COMBINED SYSTOLIC/DIASTOLIC

Patent Ductus Arteriosus

- Patent ductus arteriosus will cause continuous machinery murmur that used to radiate to the back.

- It can be close with indomethacin or high oxygen content of blood. Do not give NSAIDs to newborn. Most PDA will close by itself.

- Prostaglandin E2 is used in cyanotic congenital disease to keep the PDA open.

- PDA may also cause widened pulse pressures and bounding pulses.

Severe Coarctation of Aorta

- Coarctation of aorta produces continuous murmur.

- The systolic component is best heard at left infraclavicular (below the left scapula) region due to stenosis.

- The diastolic component is best heard over the chest wall due to blood flow through collateral vessels.

- Coarctation of aorta is often associated with Turner's syndrome (gonadal dysgenesis), an X-linked disorder with a part missing of the X-chromosome.

- Another finding of coarctation of aorta is radio-femoral delay and different blood pressures in the upper and lower extremities.

Acute Aortic Regurgitation

- Aortic regurgitation can cause a three phase murmur; mid-systolic murmur followed by S2, followed by a parasternal early diastolic and mid-diastolic murmur (Austin Flint murmur).

- Although the exact cause of an Austin Flint murmur is unknown, it is hypothesized that the mechanism of murmur is from the severe aortic regurgitation jet vibrating the anterior mitral valve leaflet, colliding with the mitral inflow during diastole, with increased mitral inflow velocity from the narrowed mitral valve orifice leading to the jet impinging on the myocardial wall.

Pathology	Valsalva maneuver/ standing	Leg raising/ squatting	Amyl nitrate/ vasodilation	Phenylephrine/ handgrip/ vasoconstriction
Hypertrophic cardiomyopathy	⇈	⇊	⇈	⇊
Mitral regurgitation, aortic regurgitation	⇊	⇈	⇊	⇈
Mitral valve Prolapse	⇈	⇊	⇈	⇊
Ventricular septal defect	⇊	⇈	⇊	⇈
Mitral stenosis	⇊	⇈	-	-
Aortic stenosis	⇊	⇈	⇈	⇊
www.medrx-education.com				

Table 3.6: change in intensity of murmurs

- **Ejection systolic:** aortic stenosis, pulmonary stenosis, hypertrophic obstructive cardiomyopathy, atrial septal defect, tetralogy of Fallot.
- **Pan-systolic:** mitral regurgitation, tricuspid regurgitation, ventricular septal defect.
- **Late systolic:** mitral valve prolapse, coarctation of aorta.
- **Early diastolic:** aortic regurgitation, pulmonary regurgitation.
- **Mid diastolic:** mitral stenosis, Austin-flint murmur (severe aortic regurgitation).

JUGULAR VENOUS PRESSURE

JVP is a measurement of right atrial pressure. Certain feature of JVP that helps to distinguish it from carotid pulse is that the JVP are:

- Non-pulsatile

- Multiphasic (waves for 1 cardiac contraction)

- Occludable (can be stopped by pressing internal Jugular vein)

- Varies with body position and respiration.

Moodley's sign: This sign is used to determine which waveform you are viewing. Feel the radial pulse while simultaneously watching the JVP. The waveform that is seen immediately after the arterial pulsation is felt is the 'v wave' of the JVP.

Kussmaul's sign: This sign describes a paradoxical rise in JVP during inspiration and is seen in constrictive pericarditis.

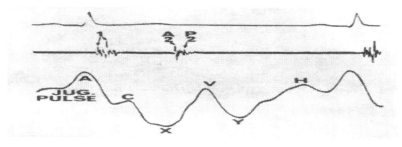

Figure 3.22: jugulovenous pressure waves*

A wave

- 'A' wave is due to atrial contraction. 'A' wave will be large if atrial pressure is high e.g. tricuspid stenosis, pulmonary stenosis, and pulmonary hypertension.

- Absent in atrial fibrillation.

- Canon 'A' wave is generated due to atrial contractions against a closed tricuspid valve. It can be seen in complete heart block, ventricular tachycardia/ectopic rhythm, nodal rhythm, and single chamber ventricular pacing.

- In type 1 heart block; 'ac' interval is prolonged.

C wave

- 'C' wave is generated in systole due to the closure of tricuspid valve.

- Some blood will be pushed back that causes a slight increase in JVP and give rise to small C wave during descent.

X-descent

- X-descent is generated due to the fall in atrial pressure during ventricular systole.

- "cv" wave or 'giant v' wave is seen in tricuspid insufficiency.

- No x-descent is seen in tricuspid insufficiency because blood is pushed back into the right atrium.

V wave

- 'V' wave is generated due to the passive filling of blood into the atrium, against a closed tricuspid valve.

Y-descent

- Y-descent is generated due to the opening of tricuspid valve and blood goes into the ventricles passively.

- In constrictive pericarditis, x-descent and y-descent falls rapidly; the y-descent is often deeper than the x-descent (Friedreich's sign).

- In pericardial tamponade, there is a loss of y-descent.

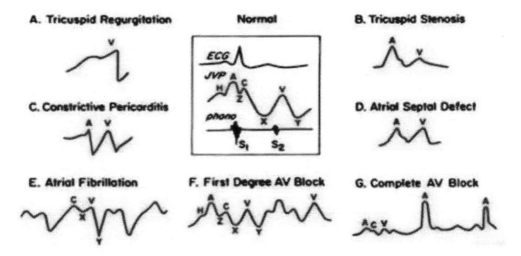

Figure 3.23: jugular venous pressure waves in various valvular pathology*

Condition	JVP waves
Tricuspid regurgitation	Large v wave (cv wave) and no x-descent
Tricuspid stenosis	Slow y-descent and elevated a wave
Pulmonary hypertension, pulmonary stenosis	Elevated a and v waves
Constrictive pericarditis	Rapid x and y descent
Cardiac tamponade	Loss of y-descent and rapid x-descent
Tension pneumothorax, superior vena cava syndrome	Distended neck veins
Atrial septal defect	Large v waves and rapid y descent
AV blocks (2nd-3rd degree)	Canon a wave
Atrial fibrillation	No a wave
AV blocks (1st degree)	Prolong a to c interval

Table 3.7: changes in Jugulovenous pressure waves

HYPERTENSION

High blood pressure is said to be present if it is persistently at or above 140/90 mmHg in adults. The higher number corresponds to systolic pressure while lower numbers correspond to diastolic pressure.

Decisions about aggressiveness of treatment are made according to the classification

CATEGORY	SYSTOLIC (mmHg)	DIASTOLIC (mmHg)
Normal	Less than 120	Less than 80
Prehypertension	120-139	80-89
Stage 1	140-159	90-99
Stage 2	160-179	100-109
Stage 3 (hypertensive crisis)	Higher than 180	Higher than 110

Table 4.1: classification of hypertension

Prehypertension is not considered abnormal, however, advise your patient for lifestyle modifications.

Primary (essential) and secondary hypertension -

- Primary (essential) hypertension is the most common cause of hypertension (95% cases). It is diagnosed when there are no identifiable secondary cause.

- Secondary hypertension is diagnosed when hypertension is due to some underlying secondary cause (5-8% cases).

PATHOGENESIS

1. Systolic Blood Pressure (SBP)

SBP correlates with stroke volume and the compliance of the aorta.

- Stroke volume is directly proportional to contractility of the heart. An increase in the contractility of the heart will cause an increase in cardiac output.

- Compliance of vessels decreases with age because of reduced elasticity of the aorta. The decrease in compliance of arteries is the mechanism for systolic hypertension in an individual >60 years of age.

- Systolic blood pressure will rise with an increase in preload, contractility, and decrease in compliance of the aorta and vice versa.

2. Diastolic Blood Pressure (DBP)

DBP correlates with the volume of blood in the aorta during diastole. Diastolic blood pressure will rise with an increase in peripheral vascular resistance, blood viscosity, and heart rate.

- DBP increases with vasoconstriction of the arterioles due to the increase in the volume of blood present in the artery during diastole.

- Increase in blood viscosity is seen in polycythemia, leukemia, dehydration while decrease in blood viscosity is seen in anemia, hyper-hydration

- Factors that constrict arteriole smooth muscle cells are α-adrenergic stimuli, catecholamine, angiotensin II, vasopressin, endothelin, and high total body sodium.

- Sodium is one of the main culprits behind hypertension. It causes fluid retention and also damages vascular endothelium producing vasoconstriction due to the release of endogenous amines.

ETIOLOGY

Primary hypertension: the most common cause of hypertension is essential hypertension (95% cases of hypertension).

- Environmental or genetic cause.
- Stress: people under stress may overeat or eat a less healthy diet, put off physical activity, drink, smoke or misuse drugs, also leads to the release of stress hormone in circulation.
- High alcohol intake
- Insulin resistance: common in obesity and is a component of 'metabolic syndrome'.
- Premature baby (low birth weight), maternal smoking and lack of breastfeeding, chewing tobacco, elevated LDL
- Obesity and lack of exercise: excess weight will increase strain on the heart, raises blood cholesterol and triglyceride levels. It will also increase the risk of diabetes. Losing as little as 10 to 20 pounds can help lower your blood pressure and your heart disease risk
- Age: greater than 55 years for men or greater than 65 years for women

Secondary Hypertension: occurs due to pre-existing pathology:

1) **Renal disease (3-5% cases)**

   - Polycystic kidney disease: multiple cysts in the kidney.

   - **Fibromuscular dysplasia** (most common in younger females): it is a developmental defect of the blood vessel wall that results in an irregular thickening of large and medium-sized arteries and thus causing a stenosis-like condition.

     Renal artery is most commonly affected which will reflexively cause activation of the renin-angiotensinogen system. Bruits can be heard due to renal artery stenosis.

     Doppler ultrasound can be used for diagnosing renal artery stenosis. Most accurate is angiogram. Treatment is renal artery angioplasty and stenting.

   - Chronic kidney disease: glomerulonephritis, diabetic nephropathy.

   - Urinary tract obstruction: kidney stones, Proteus infection (struvite stones), congenital malformations and other conditions that can obstruct the outflow.

- The renin-producing tumor will lead to high levels of renin.

- **Liddle syndrome (pseudo-hyperaldosteronism)**: severe hypertension associated with low plasma renin activity, metabolic alkalosis, hypokalemia and normal to low levels of aldosterone.

  Liddle syndrome involves abnormal kidney function, with excess reabsorption of sodium and loss of potassium and hydrogen ions from the renal tubules.

  It is treated with a combination of low sodium diet and potassium-sparing diuretic drugs.

2) **Endocrine conditions (1-2% cases)**

- Cushing's syndrome: high level of mineralocorticoids.

- Hypothyroidism

- Pheochromocytoma: tumor of the adrenal medulla which causes episodic hypertensive crisis.

- Neuroblastoma: high level of catecholamine.

- 11-hydroxylase deficiency: high level of deoxycorticosterone (acts like aldosterone) and sex hormones (hirsutism).

- Acromegaly: increase in growth hormone level in adulthood.

- Conn's syndrome: primary hyperaldosteronism resulting in hypokalemia.

3) **Vascular conditions**

- Increasing age: systolic hypertension due to decreased elasticity of the aorta in the elderly population.

- Coarctation of aorta: narrowing in the arch of the aorta will cause high blood pressure in upper extremities and low blood pressure in lower extremities. This results in under perfusion of the kidney resulting in an activation of RAS system.

- Vasculitis: inflammation of vessels (increases total peripheral resistance by narrowing vessels)

- Collagen vascular disease: occurs when problems with the immune system affect the collagen. This causes arthritis and inflammation of arteries in the tissues that connect joints and other tissues. It can be seen in ankylosing spondylitis (HLA-B27 serotype), dermatomyositis, rheumatoid arthritis (HLA-DR 3, HLA- DR 4 serotype), SLE, and other immune-mediated diseases.

4) **Epigenetic phenomena:** DNA methylation and histone modification.

- High-salt diet appears to unmask nephron development caused by methylation. Maternal water deprivation and protein restriction during pregnancy increase renin-angiotensin expression in the fetus.

- Mental stress induces a DNA methylation, which enhances autonomic responsiveness. The pattern of serine protease inhibitor gene methylation predicts preeclampsia in pregnant women.

5) **Oral contraceptives:** activates renin-angiotensinogen system because hepatic synthesis of angiotensinogen is induced by the estrogen component of oral contraceptives. The best way to manage this cause of hypertension is to stop oral contraceptives and hypertension goes away in 6 months.

6) **Exogenous steroids:** increases blood pressure by volume expansion.

7) **NSAIDs:** blocks both cyclooxygenase-1 (COX-1) and COX-2 enzymes. COX-2 has a natriuretic effect. The inhibition of COX-2 can inhibit its natriuretic effect. NSAIDs also inhibit the vasodilation effects of prostaglandins at renal afferents and produces vasoconstriction factor (endothelin-1).

8) **Neurogenic causes:** brain tumor, bulbar poliomyelitis, intracranial hypertension

9) **Drugs and toxins:** alcohol, cocaine, cyclosporine, tacrolimus, NSAIDs, erythropoietin, adrenergic medications, decongestants containing ephedrine, herbal remedies containing licorice or ephedrine.

10) **Smoking:** causes vasoconstriction and damages arteries leading to atherosclerosis, thromboangitis obliterans, Raynaud's phenomenon.

11) **Pregnancy:** gestational hypertension (new onset hypertension that develops after 20th week of pregnancy), pre-eclampsia (hypertension + proteinuria) or eclampsia (hypertension + seizures)

Smoking
Alcohol,
Steroids, ABP
OCP;
Nsmbs

CLINICAL PRESENTATION

Hypertension is usually an asymptomatic condition.

- Headache: the best evidence indicates that high blood pressure does not cause headaches except perhaps in the case of hypertensive crisis (blood pressure > 180/110 mmHg).
  According to one study, people with high blood pressure seem to have significantly fewer headaches than the general population. The higher is the pulse pressure, the stiffer is the blood vessels. In the stiffer blood vessel, there is less chance of nerve endings working properly. If the nerve endings aren't functioning correctly, there is less chance that person might feel pain.
  In other words, headache is not a reliable symptom of hypertension. Other findings that might be present in chronic hypertension are:

  - Fatigue, confusion and vision problems

  - Chest pain and difficulty breathing

  - Blood in the urine

  - Pounding in your chest, neck, or ears

  - Symptomatic nosebleeds (nose picking is most common cause of nosebleeds)

A variety of symptoms may be indirectly related to hypertension but are not always caused by it, such as:

- Blood spots in the eyes or subconjunctival hemorrhage, facial flushing and dizziness

COMPLICATION

- Left ventricular hypertrophy (most common overall complication)

- Acute myocardial infarction (most common cause of death)

- Atherosclerosis

- Intracerebral hematoma (due to rupture of Charcot-Bouchard aneurysms)

- Subarachnoid hemorrhage (due to rupture of a berry aneurysm)

- Lacunar infarcts (small infarcts due to hyaline arteriolosclerosis). Common location of lacunar infarcts includes basal ganglia, pons, internal capsule, thalamus and cerebral white matter.

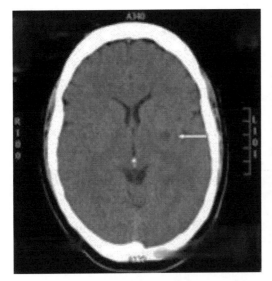 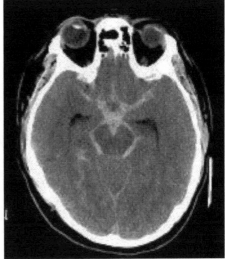

Figure 4.1: lacunar infarct of putamen*   **Figure 4.2:** subarachnoid hemorrhage*

- Benign nephrosclerosis (atrophy of tubules and sclerosis of glomeruli occurs due to hyaline arteriolosclerosis)

- Malignant hypertension (rapid increase in blood pressure accompanied by renal failure and cerebral edema)

- Hypertensive retinopathy (arteriovenous nicking, hemorrhage of retinal vessels, retinal infarction, papilledema)

MANAGEMENT

- Lifestyle modification is always the first step in the management of hypertension. It is usually recommended for 3-5 months for mild hypertension. Start medical therapy if not controlled.

- The goal of hypertension control in **diabetic hypertensive** or patient under the age of 60 **is 140/90 mmHg**. The goal of hypertension **in age greater than 60 is 150/90 mmHg.**

- The goal of antihypertensive therapy is the reduction of cardiovascular and renal morbidity and mortality, with the focus on controlling the systolic blood pressure. Most patients will achieve diastolic pressure control when the systolic blood pressure control is achieved.

- Exogenous salt intake should be limited to approximately 5 to 6 g per day.

- Body-mass index (BMI) should be reduced to 25 kg/m^2 and waist circumferences should be reduced to less than 102 cm in men and less than 88 cm in women. Decreasing the BMI is most effective way of lifestyle modification and management of hypertension.

- The patient is advised to do regular aerobic exercises and follow relaxation techniques like yoga.

- Ambulatory blood pressure monitoring should be incorporated.

- Diuretics like thiazides are the first line of drug for management of hypertension with some exceptions:

  Diabetics: ACE inhibitors are the first line of drug
  Benign prostatic hyperplasia: alpha-blockers
  Migraine headache: beta blockers, calcium channel blockers
  Pregnancy: labetalol, methyldopa, hydralazine (for acute reduction)

- For a patient whose blood pressure is more than 20 mmHg above the systolic pressure goal or more than 10 mm Hg above the diastolic pressure goal, initiation of therapy using 2 agents, one of which usually will be a thiazide diuretic, should be considered.

- If the 2 drugs combination fails to control blood pressure, add a 3rd drug. Suspect secondary hypertension if 2 or 3 drugs fail to control primary hypertension.

- Effective combination therapies include thiazide diuretics with ACE inhibitors or ARBs (angiotensin receptor blocker) or calcium blockers. calcium-channel antagonists with ARBs or ACE inhibitors. The point here is, do not combine ACE inhibitors with ARBs because of the risks of hyperkalemia, low blood pressure, and kidney failure.

- Although additional data is needed, renal denervation is a promising therapy in the treatment of resistant hypertension.

- Hypertension in pregnancy should be defined as a diastolic blood pressure of 90 mmHg or more, based on the average of at least two measurements.

- Women with a systolic blood pressure of 140 mmHg should be followed closely for development of diastolic hypertension.

- Severe hypertension is defined as a systolic pressure greater than 160 mmHg or a diastolic pressure greater than 110 mmHg.

- Chronic hypertension is the diagnosis when there is a history of elevated blood pressure before pregnancy or before 20 weeks of gestation.

- Gestational hypertension is the diagnosis when hypertension develops after 20 weeks of gestation and returns to normal baseline by 6 weeks postpartum

- Preeclampsia is the diagnosis when there is proteinuria with/without a headache, epigastric pain, pulmonary edema, and oliguria.

- In women with pre-existing hypertension, preeclampsia should be defined as resistant hypertension, new or worsening proteinuria, or one or more of the other adverse conditions.

MANAGEMENT

- Dietary salt restriction and heavy exercise are not recommended. However, strict bed rest is also not recommended usually. In-patient care should be provided for women with severe hypertension or severe pre-eclampsia.

- Blood pressure should be lowered to less than 160/110 mmHg and the goal is not to lower it significantly due to the risk of fetal hypoperfusion. Maintain systolic blood pressure at 140-150mmHg and diastolic blood pressure at 90-100mmHg.

- Best initial antihypertensive therapy is alpha-methyldopa or labetalol (best in 3rd trimester) the second line is nifedipine, and for sudden elevation of blood pressure, use hydralazine. Magnesium sulphate is not recommended.

- For women with nonsevere hypertension (140-159/90-109 mmHg) **with comorbid conditions**, antihypertensive therapy should be used to keep blood pressure below 140/90 mmHg. ACE inhibitors or ARBs should not be used due to high risk of fetal abnormalities.

- Diuretics are recommended for chronic hypertension if prescribed before gestation or if patient appears to be salt sensitive. Diuretics are not recommended in cases of preeclampsia.

HYPERTENSIVE CRISIS

CLASSIFICATION

Hypertensive crisis is divided into 2 categories:

- **Hypertensive urgency:** it is a situation where the blood pressure is greater than 180/110 mmHg, but there is no associated organ damage. Those experiencing hypertensive urgencies may or may not experience severe headache, shortness of breath, nosebleeds, and severe anxiety.

- **Hypertensive emergency:** It is characterized by acute end-organ damage which develops when blood pressure level acutely rises or when it is more than 180/120 mmHg. Acute end-organ injuries that can be seen in hypertensive emergency are:

- Hypertensive encephalopathy
- Cerebral infarction
- Subarachnoid hemorrhage
- Intracranial hemorrhage
- Myocardial ischemia/infarction,
- Acute pulmonary edema

- Aortic dissection
- Unstable angina pectoris
- Acute renal failure
- Retinopathy
- Eclampsia
- Microangiopathic hemolytic anemia

ETIOLOGY

Hypertensive crisis is a rapid unexplained rise in blood pressure in a patient with chronic essential hypertension. Most patients have a history of inadequate hypertensive treatment or an abrupt discontinuation of their medications.

Other causes of hypertensive emergencies are -

- Renal parenchymal disease: chronic pyelonephritis, primary glomerulonephritis, tubulointerstitial nephritis (accounts for 80% of all secondary causes)

- Systemic disorders with renal involvement: SLE, systemic sclerosis, vasculitis

- Renovascular disease: atherosclerotic disease, fibromuscular dysplasia, polyarteritis nodosa

- Endocrine disease: Pheochromocytoma, cushing syndrome, primary hyperaldosteronism

- Drugs: cocaine, amphetamines, cyclosporine, clonidine (withdrawal), phencyclidine, diet pills, oral contraceptive pills

- Drug interactions: monoamine oxidase inhibitors with tricyclic antidepressants, antihistamines or tyramine-containing food

- Central nervous system factors: CNS trauma or spinal cord disorders, such as Guillain-Barre syndrome

- Preeclampsia/eclampsia

CLINICAL PRESENTATION

Most common clinical presentations of hypertensive emergencies are:

- Cerebral infarction (24.5%), pulmonary edema (22.5%), hypertensive encephalopathy (16.3%), and congestive heart failure (12%)

- A severe headache and nosebleeds, altered level of consciousness and/or focal neurologic signs like loss of memory, symptoms of myocardial infarction, presentation of acute renal failure (oliguria and/or hematuria) can be present.

- Seizures can be present in pregnant women (eclampsia)

DIAGNOSIS

- Medical history

- Physical examination should include palpation of pulses in all extremities, auscultation for renal bruits, a focused neurologic examination, and a funduscopic examination

- Complete blood count and smear (to exclude a microangiopathic anemia), electrolytes, blood urea nitrogen, creatinine, urinalysis, and electrocardiogram should be obtained in all patients

- Chest X-ray in patients with shortness of breath and chest pain. Chest CT or MRI is next if chest x-ray shows evidence of widened mediastinum. [side note: transesophageal echo is not recommended in patients with aortic dissection until the blood pressure is adequately controlled]

- Head CT in patients with neurological symptoms

MANAGEMENT

- In hypertensive emergencies, the blood pressure should be lowered aggressively but do not decrease more than 25% in first hour. It should be decrease to 160/100-110 mmHg within the next 2-6 hours.

- Hypertensive urgency is usually treated with oral antihypertensive agents in an outpatient setting. For hypertensive emergency, admit the patient in ICU.

- Rapid-acting intravenous antihypertensive agents that can be used are: labetalol, esmolol, nicardipine, and sodium nitroprusside.

- Sodium nitroprusside is an extremely toxic drug and its use in the treatment of hypertensive emergencies should be avoided if possible.

- Similarly, nifedipine, nitroglycerin, and hydralazine should not be considered first-line therapies in the management of hypertensive crises because these agents are associated with significant adverse effects like end organ damage due to sudden hypotension.

THUNDERNOTE: HYPERTENSION SUBTYPES

Masked hypertension (opposite of white coat hypertension): normal blood pressure measurements at the office but elevated values elsewhere may be due to alcohol abuse or smoking.

Pseudo hypertension: It can be seen with stiff, calcified vessels in the elderly and patients with long-standing diabetes or chronic renal failure that are difficult to compress.

- The Osler maneuver (palpable radial pulse despite occlusive cuff pressure) is not a sensitive, or specific sign of pseudo- hypertension.

- Intra-arterial radial pressure measurement may be necessary for correct diagnosis.

Isolated systolic hypertension: systolic blood pressure is increased but diastolic pressure may be normal or low resulting in increased pulse pressure (the difference between systolic and diastolic pressure). Isolated systolic hypertension is often seen in older people. It can be explained by increased arterial stiffness, which typically accompanies aging and may be exacerbated by high blood pressure.

PULMONARY HYPERTENSION

Pulmonary hypertension is defined as mean pulmonary arterial pressure >25mmHg at rest.

> 25

ETIOLOGY

- Idiopathic (occurs due to intimal fibrosis and replacement of normal endothelial structure due to some unknown reason. Genetic mutation in BMPR gene is seen in 15% cases of idiopathic pulmonary hypertension)
- Chronic lung disease (COPD)
- Secondary to left heart disease (low ejection fraction, signs of pulmonary edema)
- Thromboembolism (due to recurrent thromboembolism, sudden onset of shortness of breath can be seen)

CLINICAL PRESENTATION

SOB, tachy
systolic murmur

- Progressive shortness of breath
- Systolic murmur at the left sternal border that increases with inspiration (tricuspid regurgitation)
- Peripheral edema
- Tachycardia, pleuritic chest pain

DIAGNOSIS

- ECG is done to assess myocardial infarction
- Echocardiogram is done to assess valvular pathology and pulmonary systolic arterial pressure
- In hemodynamically stable patients, exclude pulmonary thromboembolism and interstitial lung disease. Perform pulmonary function test to check lung pathology. If abnormal, evaluate with chest CT scan. If normal, perform V/Q scan. If perfusion defects are present, perform spiral CT or pulmonary angiography.
- Cardiac catheterization is the most accurate test but rarely done if necessary.

MANAGEMENT

- Lifestyle modifications such as exercise improves long-term outcomes improving peak oxygen consumption in all patients with pulmonary hypertension.
- Pulmonary hypertension secondary to left systolic dysfunction: loop diuretics and ACE inhibitors, often with beta blockers, and in some cases spironolactone.
- Pulmonary hypertension due to chronic lung disease: home oxygen therapy with or without bronchodilator therapy.
- Idiopathic pulmonary hypertension: bosentan (endothelin receptor blocker), sildenafil (PDE-5 inhibitor), and/or epoprostenol (prostaglandin I_2)
- Pulmonary hypertension due to thromboembolism: long-term anticoagulation with warfarin.

ARTERIOSCLEROSIS

Arteriosclerosis means hardening of arteries due to thickening of vessel wall and classified into 3 categories

MONCKEBERG MEDIAL SCLEROSIS

- Monkenberg arteriosclerosis is also called as medial calcific sclerosis.

- It can occur in the elderly population (1% prevalence) and in diabetics.

- It is usually more benign than other forms of arteriosclerosis because it does not cause narrowing of the lumen.

PATHOGENESIS

- Calcium deposits are found in the muscular layer (tunica media) of medium-sized arteries like femoral, radial, ulnar, and tibial artery.

- Monkenberg arteriosclerosis is an example of dystrophic calcification.

CLINICAL PRESENTATION

- An individual is usually asymptomatic unless severe. However, if severe, it is a poor prognostic sign for diabetics and heart patients due to the stiffening of vessel.

DIAGNOSIS

- Usually detected incidentally on x-ray or mammogram or biopsy.
- Seen as an opaque vessel on normal x-rays and purple calcium deposits on histological slides.

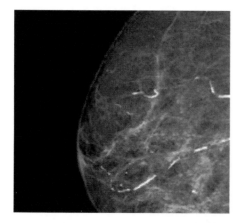

Figure 4.3: Monkenberg medial sclerosis on mammogram

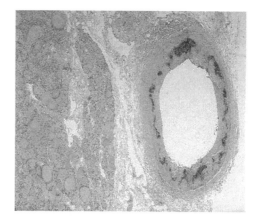

Figure 4.4: dark blue color surrounding the lumen are calcium deposits.

THUNDERNOTE: Dystrophic Calcification and Metastatic Calcification

DYSTROPHIC CALCIFICATION

- Calcification occurs in degenerated/necrotic tissue, hyalinized scars, degenerated foci in leiomyoma and caseous nodules.
- It occurs as a reaction to tissue damage.
- Blood calcium level is usually normal.
- Dystrophic calcification is a localized process.

METASTATIC CALCIFICATION

- Deposition of calcium occurs in normal tissue, because of an increase in the level of calcium.
- It can occur because of a defect in metabolism or increased absorption or decreased excretion of calcium and related minerals, as seen in hyperparathyroidism.
- Metastatic calcification is a generalized process (multiple tissues can be affected at one time).
- It typically involves interstitial tissues, especially of kidney, lung, gastric mucosa and vasculature.

ARTERIOLOSCLEROSIS

- Arteriosclerosis means hardening of arterioles

CLASSIFICATION

- Hyaline arteriolosclerosis
- Hyperplastic arteriolosclerosis

	Hyaline arteriolosclerosis	Hyperplastic arteriolosclerosis
Causes	Diabetes, chronic hypertension**, aging	Malignant hypertension (sudden rise in blood pressure)
Histology	Pink, glassy arterial wall thickening with luminal narrowing.	"Onion skin" appearance (concentric wall thickening)
Mechanism	Due to increase in protein deposition in the vessel wall which leads to narrowing of the lumen.	Due to duplication of basement membrane and smooth muscle hyperplasia in the arterioles.

Table 4.2: difference between hyaline and hyperplastic arteriolosclerosis

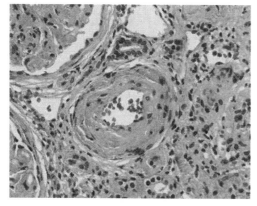

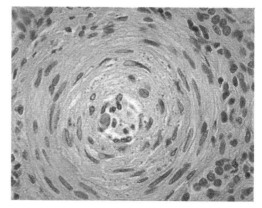

Figure 4.5: Hyaline Arteriolosclerosis **Figure 4.6:** Hyperplastic Arteriolosclerosis

**Diabetes mellitus will cause non-enzymatic glycosylation of the basement membrane of arterioles. This leads to leakage of protein from the plasma into the vessel wall.

In diabetes, both renal afferent and efferent arterioles are commonly affected while in hypertension, afferent renal arterioles are more commonly affected).

High blood pressure in the arterioles causes extravasation of proteins into the vessel wall.

Hyperplastic arteriolosclerosis

- In malignant hypertension, these hyperplastic changes are often accompanied by fibrinoid necrosis of arterial intima and media.

- These changes are more prominent in the kidney and can lead to ischemia and acute renal failure.

ATHEROSCLEROSIS

PATHOGENESIS

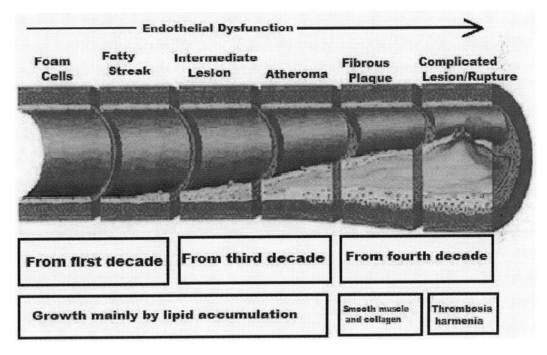

Figure 4.7: formation of atheromatous plaque

- **Endothelial cell injury** is the first step in the pathogenesis of atherosclerosis.
- After the endothelial injury, infiltration of macrophage in the intima and platelet adherence to damaged endothelium will occur.
- The next step in pathogenesis is the release of various inflammatory mediators like cytokines and growth factors, which results in hyperplasia of smooth muscle cells. The proliferation of smooth muscle cells and macrophage will also occur and the debris accumulates in the intima.
- Cholesterol (carried by LDL) enters into this macrophage and forms a large cell called foam cell. This will lead to the formation of fatty streak, which is commonly found at very young age in the general population. The fatty streaks are not considered pathologic.

- After the formation of fatty streak, HDL will come and take up the cholesterol debris and deliver it to the liver. LDL will carry modified form of cholesterol back to the body tissues from the liver and cycle continues.

Normally, this cycle is well controlled, however when there are imbalances or enzymatic reactions between HDL and LDL due to various stressors, this will result in the accumulation of cholesterol and further development into atheromatous plaque.

- Smooth muscle cells and macrophage will release various components of extracellular matrix like proteoglycans, collagen, elastin, metalloproteinase, thromboxane A2, platelet derived growth factors and other mediators into the atheroma.
- These components will result in the formation of fibrous cap surrounding this debris. The necrotic cells along with foam cells generally accumulate in the center of atheroma. This is the primary lesion of atherosclerosis.
- Plaque can rupture and lead to vessel thrombosis. The necrotic core is exposed to the endothelial surface which then serve as a nidus for the formation of thrombus.
- Dystrophic calcification and ulceration in plaque can occur at later stages.

THUNDERNOTE: FAMILIAL HYPERCHOLESTEROLEMIA

- Familial hypercholesterolemia is an autosomal dominant condition (50% probability that a newborn will have a disease if one of the parents has dominant gene).
- LDL receptor deficiency on the liver results in increased amount of circulating LDL cholesterol along with de-novo synthesis. This results in an increase in delivery of cholesterol to the intima of vessel and oxidation which results in atheromatous plaque formation.
- Xanthoma at Achilles' tendon is diagnostic. Xanthelasma is a yellow plaque on the eyelid.
- Individual will have a high risk of premature coronary artery disease and stroke.

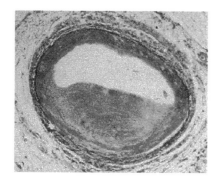

Figure 4.8: Narrowing of the lumen due to atherosclerotic process.

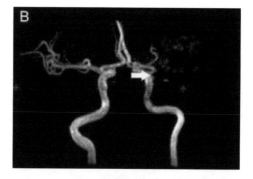

Figure 4.9: MRI angiography of cerebral vessels shows the left middle cerebral artery thrombosis.

RISK FACTORS

- Hypertension: hypertension will accelerate atherosclerosis by producing endothelial cell dysfunction. Renal artery atherosclerosis may activate the renin-angiotensin-aldosterone system and further worsen hypertension.
- Diabetes mellitus: diabetes will increase non-enzymatic glycosylation of endothelium.
- Cigarette smoking
- Infections like Chlamydia pneumonia.
- Toxins and metabolic problems like elevated homocysteine, hyperlipidemias, and oxidized LDL.
- Functional change in endothelium due to increased oxidative stress or abnormalities in coagulation or platelets
- Obesity, lack of exercise, family history (multiple genes)

SITE OF INVOLVEMENT

- Abdominal aorta (most common)
- Coronary artery (2nd most common)
- Popliteal artery
- Internal carotid artery

COMPLICATION

Long-term effects of atherosclerosis depend on which arteries are blocked:

LAD

- Coronary artery disease: left anterior descending artery is more commonly affected than the right coronary artery. Narrowing will result in angina or acute myocardial infarction on plaque rupture.

- Carotid artery disease: narrowing of the internal carotid artery, middle cerebral artery more commonly results in transient ischemic attacks or stroke.

- Peripheral artery disease: narrowing of arteries in the arms or leg will produce symptoms like claudication, slow healing of wounds, foot ulcers, cool skin temperature, diminished hair-nail growth in extremities, and diminished pedal pulse. Bruits can be present. In rare cases, poor circulation in the arms or legs can cause tissue death (gangrene).

- Aneurysms: most people with aneurysms have no symptoms. Pain and throbbing in the area of an aneurysm may occur and is a medical emergency. If an aneurysm bursts, life-threatening internal bleeding will occur.

DIAGNOSIS

Ankle Brachial index <0.9

- The ankle-brachial index ratio < 0.9 is consistent with the peripheral arterial disease. If the patient has claudication and ABI is normal, then suspect disease in small vessels.
- Angiography is the most accurate diagnostic test.

MANAGEMENT

- Control the risk factors for peripheral artery disease. Stop smoking and follow routine exercise schedule for development of collateral circulation. If patient develops pain at rest or have an impact on a lifestyle where he/she has to stop walking every other block, then there is a risk of gangrene and it should be managed surgically.
- Aspirin (best initial therapy), cilostazol (platelet aggregation inhibitor)
- Angioplasty and stenting for short stenotic segments for severe disease. Bypass graft or longer stents for the more extensive disease can be done.
- Statins are indicated if LDL level is greater than 100 mg/dl.

THUNDERNOTE: ACUTE PERIPHERAL ARTERY OCCLUSION

Cause:
- Rupture and thrombosis of an atherosclerotic plaque
- Embolus from the heart or thoracic or abdominal aorta
- Aortic dissection
- Acute compartment syndrome

Clinical presentation:

- **Pain:** pain or cramps that develop with increased walking or exercise (claudication)
- **Pallor:** progress from pale to a mottled cyanosis
- **Paresthesia:** altered sensations, serious consequences if it rapidly progresses
- **Paralysis:** weakness on dorsiflexion of foot or toe (peroneal nerve distribution)
- **Pulse:** absent or weak pulse below the area of occlusion, cold skin

Diagnosis:
- Clinical diagnosis. Immediate angiography is required to confirm location of the occlusion and guide therapy.
- Duplex ultrasonography can be done to check the resolution and blood flow after an initiation of thrombolytic.

Management:
- Thrombolysis with tissue plasminogen activator or urokinase (in acute occlusion of less than 2 weeks), or bypass surgery.
- Embolectomy (catheter or surgical) is done when there are contraindications for thrombolysis.
- Fasciotomy is indicated for compartment syndrome.

LERICHE SYNDROME

- Acute or chronic peripheral aortoiliac occlusion

Cause: atherosclerosis (most common cause), vasculitis

Clinical presentation: claudication, absent/weak femoral pulse and erectile dysfunction.

Diagnosis: CT angiography (best diagnostic test), Contrast MRA if CT is not possible

Management: Bypass surgery or balloon angioplasty with/without stent implantation is done to relieve the obstruction.

MIDAORTIC SYNDROME

- A similar presentation like peripheral artery disease, but very rare and different pathophysiology. It occurs due to the narrowing of the abdominal aorta and its branches without atherosclerosis or vasculitis. Exact cause is unknown. Aortic bifurcation and iliac artery are spared. Occlusion is at mid-aortic level that also causes renal failure and hypertension along with intermittent claudication.

- **Management:** Balloon angioplasty with a stent to expand the lumen of the aorta, fenestrated graft with implantation of renal arteries.

THUNDERNOTE: Calciphylaxis

- Calciphylaxis is also called calcific uremic arteriolopathy.

- It is generally seen in the last stage of chronic kidney disease.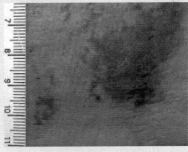

- Calciphylaxis results in chronic non-healing wounds and is usually fatal. Calciphylaxis is a rare but serious condition.

- Extraskeletal calcifications are also observed in some patients with hypercalcemic states, including patients with the milk-alkali syndrome, sarcoidosis, primary hyperparathyroidism, and hypervitaminosis D.

- Patients with calciphylaxis have small vessel calcification and a netlike pattern of calcifications and may result in end-organ necrosis.

- Aneurysms are localized dilation and outpouching from the vessel wall.
- They can be due to congenital causes or acquired.
- Aneurysms are mainly due to the weakness of tunica media

TYPE	ETIOLOGY	LOCATION	Features
Abdominal aortic aneurysm	Atherosclerosis (most common), Due to the defect in the connective tissue, familial.	Below the renal artery orifices	Usually asymptomatic, but bruits can be heard if renal or visceral artery is compressed. Pulsatile epigastric mass can be felt sometimes. Rupture causes sudden severe left flank pain and hypotension due to the blood loss in the retroperitoneum
Thoracic aortic aneurysm	Due to the cystic medial degeneration or atherosclerosis (look for abdominal aortic aneurysm)	Ascending and descending aorta (distal to origin of subclavian artery)	Usually asymptomatic but it can compress surrounding structures like recurrent laryngeal nerve (hoarseness) and produce associated symptoms. CT and aortography are the investigations of choice. X-Rays are nonspecific.
Berry (saccular) aneurysm	Hypertension, coarctation of aorta, atherosclerosis, congenital, polycystic kidney disease	Circle of Willis (most common site is at the junction of anterior communicating branch with anterior cerebral artery)	Berry aneurysm rupture will cause subarachnoid hemorrhage. Patient often presents complaining of sudden onset of severe occipital headache, and nuchal rigidity. Rx: Immediate surgical repair. Fusiform aneurysms (giant brain aneurysms) involves the whole segment of the artery.
Mycotic aneurysm	Salmonella species (50%) S. aureus (38%).	Femoral artery (38%) is most common site followed by abdominal aorta (30%)	Vessel wall weakening due to an infection that invades vessel. Patient presents with fever, leukocytosis (+/-) with back pain/palpable aneurysm. Surgery is almost always required.

Syphilitic aneurysm	T. pallidum (tertiary syphilis)	Aortic arch (ascending and transverse arch)	T. pallidum infects vasa vasorum and causes vasculitis; endarteritis obliterans. Plasma cell infiltrates vessel wall and may decrease the size of arterial lumen. Involvement of the aortic root can cause aortic regurgitation.
Micro-aneurysm or Charcot-Bouchard aneurysm	Hypertension, diabetes mellitus	Striatal branch of middle cerebral artery which supplies basal ganglia	Rupture causes intracerebral hemorrhage; hemorrhagic shock (sudden loss of sensation or paralysis).

Table 4.3: characteristics of different kinds of aneurysms

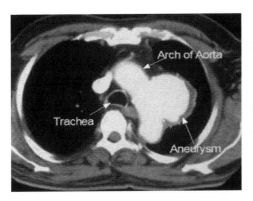

Figure 4.10: thoracic aortic aneurysm*

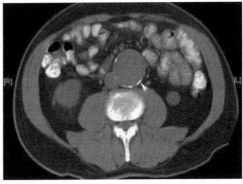

Figure 4.11: abdominal aortic aneurysm*

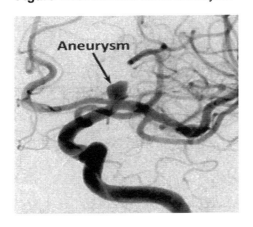

Figure 4.12: berry aneurysm*

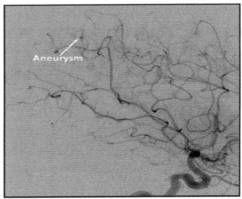

Figure 4.13: Mycotic aneurysm*

ABDOMINAL AORTIC ANEURYSM SCREENING

Screening with ultrasound is recommended only in high-risk groups. Screening in such high risk groups has shown to reduce mortality rate by 43%.

High-risk group includes but not limited to:

- Men > 65 years of age who have long-term history of smoking.
- Men > 55 years of age who have family history of abdominal aortic aneurysm.
- Women > 55 years who have both smoking history and family history.
- Screening is not recommended for a woman of any age who does not have smoking and family history.

MANAGEMENT

Indication for repair: abdominal aneurysm greater than 5.5 cm or growth > 1 cm/year, thoracic aneurysm greater than 6.5 or growth > 1 cm/year.

Aortic Diameter	Recommendation
Less than 3.0cm	No further testing or screening
3.0 to 3.9cm	Re-test with abdominal ultrasound at 3 years after initial screening, then every 3 years until age 75
4.0-4.9cm	Re-test with abdominal ultrasound at 6 months after initial screening, then annually until age 75
5.0 cm or greater	Retest with abdominal ultrasound at 6 months after initial screening, then annually until age 75. Refer patient to vascular surgery if aneurysm is expanding or diameter greater than 5.5cm.

Table 4.4: management of abdominal aortic aneurysm

- Aortic dissection is an intimal tear with dissection of blood through media of the aortic wall. As the tear extends along the wall of the aorta, blood can flow between the layers of aortic wall.
- It more often occurs in the proximal aorta due to the high stress generated by the force of cardiac output.

PATHOGENESIS

- Aortic dissection occurs due to the preexisting weakness of the tunica media.
- The possible reason for medial wall weakness is cystic medial degeneration in which elastic tissues are fragmented in the media and leads to accumulation of degraded matrix material.

ETIOLOGY

- Aging, hypertension, atherosclerosis

- Blunt trauma to the chest, such as hitting the steering wheel of a car during an accident

- Bicuspid aortic valve, coarctation of aorta

- Connective tissue disorders like Marfan's syndrome

- Heart surgery or procedures

- Pregnancy, arteritis, and syphilis

4 bony injuries that can cause aortic dissection are;

- Sternal fracture

- 1st rib fracture

- Scapular fractures

- Flail chest

Suspect aortic dissection if the chest x-ray shows widened mediastinum following mediastinal injuries.

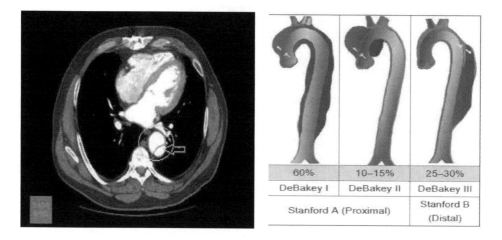

Figure 4.14: CT showing aortic dissection, **Figure 4.15:** types of aortic dissection

CLINICAL PRESENTATION

- Acute aortic dissection is characterized by sudden severe sharp anterior chest pain that radiates to the back.

- Some patients can feel pain migrating downward through the aorta. Chronic dissections can be asymptomatic.

Type A Dissection

- Type A aortic dissection occurs at the root of the aorta.

- If it grows anteriorly, it can occlude aortic branches going to head and neck. If grows backward, it can cause cardiac tamponade, or aortic valve dysfunction (aortic insufficiency) or can block the coronary artery (arises from aortic sinus, behind the aortic valves) leading to myocardial infarction and death.

- Cerebrovascular accidents or pseudo-hypotension (compression of subclavian artery) can occur if the dissection occlude aortic branches.

Type B dissection

- Type B dissection occurs after the branching of subclavian artery.

- No aortic branches going to head, neck and arm are affected and therefore, neurological deficit, cardiac dysfunction, and pseudo-hypotension will be absent. It often grows downward and can cause narrowing of vessels that come across its path (renal artery stenosis) or superior mesenteric arteries (mesenteric ischemia).

COMPLICATION

- Rupture (most commonly in pericardial sac followed by pleural cavity and peritoneum) and hypotension

- Aortic regurgitation (in 2/3rd Case)

- Myocardial infarction (3%)

- Pericardial tamponade (most common cause of death)

DIAGNOSIS

- History, CT angiogram (most accurate) or transesophageal echocardiogram (when there are contraindications for CT angiogram or in an emergency setting when suspicion for aortic dissection are high. Do not perform transesophageal echocardiogram in aortic dissection with hypertensive crisis).

- Chest x-ray will show mediastinal widening but is very nonspecific, however, it is the best initial test to do on suspect and if widened; beta-blockers (labetalol, esmolol), nifedipine and nitroglycerine can be given if blood pressure is high.

MANAGEMENT

- On suspect of aortic dissection, the best initial step in management is to reduce the blood pressure with esmolol or labetalol, and nitroglycerine.

- In medical management targeted mean blood pressure is 65-70 mmHg or the lowest blood pressure tolerated by the patient.

- Beta blockers (esmolol, labetalol) are the drug of choice followed by nitroglycerine.

- For Stanford type A aortic dissection, surgery is superior to medical management.

- For uncomplicated Stanford type B dissections (including abdominal aortic dissections), medical management is preferred over surgical.

- Surgery is indicated if the diameter of pseudo-lumen is > 5.5 cm.

THUNDERNOTE: FLAIL CHEST

Flail chest is defined as fracture of 2 or more adjacent ribs at 2 different points on each rib.

Flail chest can cause paradoxical bleeding, chest pain, pneumothorax with or without hemothorax, pulmonary contusion, cardiac contusion (causes arrhythmia and death) and aortic dissection.

The patient is emergently managed by placing chest tube on both sides of the lung at 5th intercostal space on anterior axillary line, then do positive pressure ventilation. Adjust the ventilator setting to avoid high pressure associated lung trauma.

Pain is controlled by epidural anesthesia. Nerve block is appropriate when only 1 rib is fractured but flail chest have multiple rib fractures.

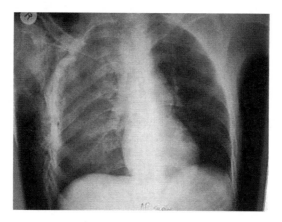

Figure 4.16: Right-sided multiple rib fractures and flail chest, right pulmonary contusion and subcutaneous emphysema.

COARCTATION OF AORTA

Coarctation of aorta is the narrowing of the aortic segment. Coarctation of aorta presents early in life with congestive heart failure or later in life with hypertension

CLASSIFICATION

- Congenital form: narrowing is prior to ligamentum arteriosus (pre-ductal).

- Adult form: narrowing is distal to ligamentum arteriosus (post-ductal). In adults, it is usually associated with bicuspid aortic valve, turner syndrome, and patent ductus arteriosus.

CLINICAL PRESENTATION

Neonates

- Coarctation of aorta is due to the medial wall thickening in a segment of aorta. It can develop into congestive heart failure.

- The abrupt closure of patent ductus arteriosus in severe coarctation will cause sudden rise in left heart pressure. The high pressure in the left heart will result in backward high pressure in pulmonary circulation. This will acutely develop in pulmonary edema. If the foramen ovale is not closed or if the atrial septal defect is present, it will cause right ventricular failure due to increase in amount of circulating blood. Cardiomegaly and right sided hypertrophy is seen on radiological findings.

- Young patients may present in the first few weeks of life with poor feeding, tachypnea, lethargy and progress to overt congestive heart failure and shock.

- Newborn may appear well prior to hospital discharge if patent ductus arteriosus is not closed. The deterioration coincides with the closure of the patent ductus arteriosus.

Adults

- Blood flow will increase in the aortic branches that originates prior to the narrowing, but it decreases distal to the narrowing. This results in high blood pressure in upper extremity and low blood pressure in the lower extremities (>10mmHg difference).

- Another finding of coarctation of aorta include claudication in the lower extremities with prolonged continuous walking.

- Low pressure distal to the narrowing will cause activation of RAAS system due to low renal perfusion. This will further increase blood pressure and the condition deteriorates. In some cases, renin level will be normal.

- Due to high pressure in the upper body, collateral vessels are formed between the internal thoracic subclavian artery and aorta. Some amount of blood will flow from ascending aorta to internal thoracic artery to the descending aorta and maintains perfusion distal to the narrowing.

- Other presenting symptoms may include headaches, chest pain, fatigue, or even life-threatening intracranial hemorrhage due to the rupture of a berry aneurysm.

DIAGNOSIS

- In neonates, sepsis and congestive heart failure will have a similar presentation. Blood analysis, urine, and cerebrospinal fluid cultures, electrolyte levels, BUN, creatinine, arterial blood gas, serum lactate level and glucose concentrations must be checked to exclude sepsis.

- In adults, there is blood pressure discrepancy between the upper and lower extremity. Chest x-ray will show rib notching below the ribs due to continuous high-pressure pulsation in intercostal arteries.

- Echocardiography is a most specific test for all congenital heart disease in neonates.

- Laboratory studies in older patients who present with hypertension include urinalysis, electrolyte levels, BUN, creatinine, and glucose concentrations.

- MRI and CT are useful in older or postoperative patients to assess residual arch obstruction, arch hypoplasia, or formation of aneurysms.

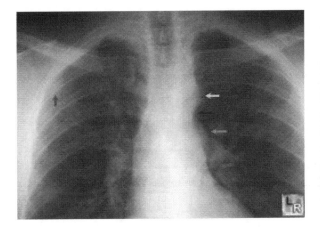 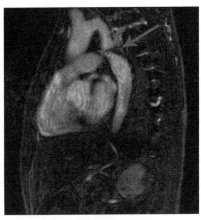

Image 4.17: Rib notching (bilateral red arrows), aortic knob (upper yellow arrow), coarctation (central blue arrow), post aortic dilation (lower green arrow)*

Image 4.18: MRA showing coarctation of aorta*

MANAGEMENT

- If the neonate is unstable, first step is to stabilize the neonate with diuretics and prostaglandin E2 (to prevent closure of ductus arteriosus) and then perform surgery.

- In adults, if the narrowing is mild, surgery is usually not required. Manage with antihypertensive therapy like beta-blockers and diuretics (best initial therapy).

- ACEi/ARBs are not indicated because they will result in severe hypotension in the lower extremity.

- Surgical correction is indicated if left ventricular dysfunction has developed or patient's condition is deteriorating.

Coarctation of aorta → NO ACE/ARB

VASCULITIS

Vasculitis is an inflammation of the blood vessel wall.

CLASSIFICATION

- **Large vessel vasculitis:** involves the aorta and it's major branches; e.g. giant cell arteritis, and Takayasu arteritis

- **Medium vessel vasculitis:** involves muscular arteries; e.g. polyarteritis nodosa, Kawasaki disease, and thromboangitis obliterans.

- **Small vessel vasculitis:** involves arterioles and capillaries; e.g. Granulomatosis with polyangitis (formerly known as Wegner's granulomatosis), microscopic polyangitis, Churg-Strauss syndrome.

VASCULITIS	PATHOGENESIS	CLINICAL PRESENTATION	DIAGNOSIS AND MANAGEMENT
Temporal giant cell arteritis	Segmental granulomatous inflammation involving branches of carotid artery Females > 50 years of age are more commonly affected	**Headache** (temporal a.), **visual disturbances** (ophthalmic a., usually unilateral), **jaw claudication, fever**, myalgia (proximal stiffness) It is associated with polymyalgia rheumatica (normal creatinine kinase, elevated ESR)	ESR >60mm/hr (best first step). If ESR is <60mm/hr, think about another pathology. If ESR is >60mm/hr, immediate high-dose prednisolone is indicated to prevent irreversible vision loss. Multinucleated giant cells and intimal fibrosis on biopsy (taken from multiple segments).
Takayasu pulseless arteritis	Granulomatous inflammation involving arch of aorta at branching points.	Visual disturbances, neurological symptoms due to diminished blood flow, fever. arthritis, myalgia.	ESR >50mm/hr, blood pressure in legs may be >10mmHg than upper extremities. Angiography is gold standard. Biopsy plays little to no role in

	Young Asian females < 50 years of age are more commonly affected.	Absent or weak pulse in upper extremities, transient ischemic attacks	diagnosis. Rx is high-dose prednisolone followed by long term low-dose prednisolone.
Polyarteritis nodosa	Characterized by transmural inflammation with fibrinoid necrosis, Multiple organs are involved EXCEPT pulmonary arteries. Mediated by immune complex (type III hypersensitivity) if associated with Hepatitis B i.e. in 30% cases.	More commonly seen in young adults. **foot/wrist drop**, **hypertension** (due to renal artery involvement), **abdominal pain** with **melena** (due to mesenteric artery involvement), acute myocardial infarction (if coronary a. involved), fever, weight loss, headache, skin nodules	Angiography is the best initial diagnostic test. Confirm it with biopsy of skin, symptomatic nerve or muscle. Multiple lesions are at different stage of development. As the lesion heals by fibrosis it will produce a string of pearl appearance on imaging. Rx: high-dose corticosteroids **and** cyclophosphamide.
Kawasaki Disease	It involves medium-sized muscular artery including coronary arteries. An inflammation that spreads completely around the coronary artery; the artery then begins to dilate and may form aneurysm.	It is seen more commonly in Asian children < 4 years of age. Unexplained fever >5 days, rash on palm and soles, dry lips, conjunctivitis, strawberry (red) tongue and cervical lymphadenitis (least common).	Diagnosis is clinical, exclude other infectious causes of fever. Coronary artery involvement can cause aneurysm rupture, thrombosis with MI. The primary goal in management is to prevent cardiac complications. Rx: admit the patient to the hospital; IVIG with aspirin.

Thromboangitis obliterans	It is an inflammatory endarteritis that causes vaso-occlusive phenomenon. It involves small and medium-sized arteries and is limited to tunica intima. Legs are always involved. **It is associated with smoking.**	It is more common in young males in Jews, Indians and Koreans. **Claudication** is the first manifestation. Complications like ulcers, gangrene and auto-amputation of fingers and toes can develop if blood flow is severely compromised. It can involve neural components and vein (phlebitis)	Diagnosis is clinical Rx: smoking cessation is best first and last step in management. Prostaglandins, alpha blockers, nifedipine, or pentoxyfilline can be considered but. pharmacological therapy is generally ineffective and endovascular revascularization is not possible.
Granulomatosis with polyangitis (Wegner's granulomatosis)	Necrotizing granulomatous inflammation and pauci-immune vasculitis in small and medium-sized vessels.	It generally affects male 25-50 years of age. Involves nasopharynx (**sinusitis**, saddle nose), lungs (**hemoptysis**) and kidneys (**hematuria** due to rapidly progressive glomerulonephritis)	Presence of c-ANCA against proteinase-3 is most specific. Large nodular densities on chest x-ray. Rx: cyclophosphamide with high-dose steroids. If creatinine level > 5.65mg/dl, plasmapheresis is indicated. Relapse is common; long-term maintenance therapy with azathioprine or methotrexate is considered.

Microscopic polyangiitis (leukocytoclastic angiitis)	Pauci-immune, Non-granulomatous necrotizing vasculitis that involves arterioles, capillary and venules. Upper respiratory track is spared.	Though rare, it is more common in white males > 50 years of age. Fever, malaise, fatigue, weight loss, hematuria, skin rash (including ulceration) and arthralgia (similar presentation like granulomatosis with polyangitis).	ANCA positive (either p-ANCA or c-ANCA positive). Biopsy of affected organ system is gold standard. It may show infiltration with fragmented neutrophils with or without fibrinoid necrosis. Rx: cyclophosphamide and prednisolone.
Churg-Strauss Syndrome	Granulomatous small vessel vasculitis with asthma (increase in eosinophil count and IgE level)	Lungs and heart are more commonly involved, asthma, sinusitis. Wrist & foot drop can occur due to peripheral nerve involvement (mono neuritis multiplex)	CBC shows eosinophilia, anemia. p-ANCA positive in 40% cases, elevated serum IgE level Rx: steroids alone are adequate..
Henoch-Schonlein Purpura	IgA mediated small vessel vasculitis. IgA complexes deposits in renal mesangium and vessel walls. It usually occurs after upper respiratory or GI infection.	It is the most common vasculitis in children <18 years of age. Fever, headache, and anorexia followed by palpable purpura on the buttocks and legs (hallmark finding), abdominal pain and melena, polyarthritis (knee and ankle), hematuria	Clinical diagnosis, exclude other diagnosis and renal function test. Rx: hydration, NSAIDs or steroids for joint pain or nephritis. Hospitalize if severe abdominal pain and melena, monitor renal function. Avoid NSAIDs if creatinine is high.

Table 4.5: Vasculitis*

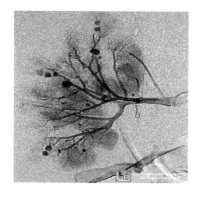

Figure 4.19: angiogram of polyarteritis nodosa*

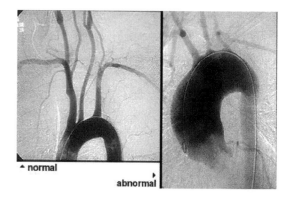

Figure 4.20: angiogram of Takayasu arteritis*

THUNDERNOTE: CRYOGLOBULINEMIA

A large amount of circulating cryoglobulins in the blood precipitate at low temperature and more commonly involves the kidney. It is associated with:

- Multiple myelomas (10-15% cases)

- SLE, rheumatoid arthritis (25-30% cases); due to IgM-IgG complexes; looks like rheumatoid factors

- Hepatitis C infection (50-60% cases)

- Mycoplasma pneumonia and certain leukemia

Clinical presentation: cryoglobulinemia due to hepatitis C or connective tissue disease will have a similar presentation like vasculitis; purpura, arthralgia, myalgia, and fatigue. Cryoglobulinemia due to malignancy like multiple myeloma will have hyperviscosity syndrome.

Diagnosis: serum cryoglobulins level, rule out hepatitis C and multiple myeloma.

Management: treat the underlying cause, corticosteroids and/or cyclophosphamide are indicated upon evidence of end-organ involvement such as renal damage or progressive neurological findings. Plasmapheresis for severe life-threatening findings.

RAYNAUD PHENOMENON

Raynaud phenomenon is an excessive reduction of the blood flow in response to cold or emotional stress, causing discoloration of the fingers, toes and occasionally other areas. It can be part of:

- Raynaud's disease (primary Raynaud's phenomenon)

- Raynaud's syndrome (secondary Raynaud's phenomenon)

A careful medical history will often reveal whether the condition is primary or secondary. Once this has been established, an examination is largely to identify or exclude possible secondary causes.

CLINICAL PRESENTATION

- **Pallor:** when exposed to cold temperatures, the blood supply to the fingers or toes, and in some cases the nose or earlobes, is markedly reduced; the skin turns pale or white and becomes cold and numb.
- **Cyanosis:** when the oxygen supply is depleted, the skin color turns blue
- **Rubor and pain:** these events are episodic, and when the episode subsides or the area is warmed; the blood flow returns and the skin color first turns red, and then back to normal, often accompanied by swelling, tingling, and a painful "pins and needles" sensation.

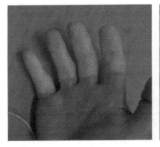 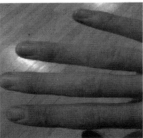 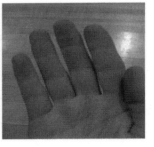

Figure 4.21: pallor, cyanosis, and rubor*

	Primary	Secondary
Onset	Younger age especially women	Older age (> 30 years)
Symptoms	Mild (absence of tissue necrosis, ulceration, or gangrene. Smoking and caffeine can worsen the symptoms	Episodes are intense, painful and may be associated with ischemic lesions. Additionally, symptoms of underlying pathology might also exist.
Autoimmune disease test results	Negative (because no underlying cause)	Positive (elevated ESR, ANA, rheumatoid factor, autoantibodies)
History	Migraine headache, prinzmetal's angina	SLE, scleroderma, Sjogren syndrome, thromboangitis obliterans, beta-blockers and other connective tissue diseases.

Table 4.6: primary and secondary Raynaud's phenomenon

MANAGEMENT

- Best initial management is a lifestyle modification that includes avoidance of cold exposure, smoking cessation, avoidance of sympathomimetic drugs.

- For stable condition: use topical nitrates or long- acting calcium channel blockers (nifedipine)

- For unstable condition (more common with secondary Raynaud; ischemia and ulcers): use nifedipine/nitrates with aspirin/heparin. Phosphodiesterase V inhibitors can be used off-label.

- Prevent the digital ulcers with bosentan in patients with systemic sclerosis, PDE-V Inhibitors (off-label).

THUNDERNOTE CREST SYNDROME

CREST Syndrome (limited cutaneous form of systemic sclerosis)

C = Calcinosis (thickening and tightening of skin due to calcium deposition)

R = Raynaud's phenomenon (1st manifestation)

E = Oesophageal dysmotility (dysphagia in mid-lower esophagus)

S = Sclerodactyly (thickening of skin of fingers distal to metacarpophalangeal joints. It can complicate into ulcers, due to fibrosis.

T = Telangiectasia (more common with scleroderma-related vascular disease, dilated capillaries on the skin of the face, palmar surface of hands and mucous membranes.

Diagnosis: clinical diagnose, anti-centromere antibodies.

Scleroderma (diffuse form of systemic sclerosis)

Scleroderma affects the internal organs also (other than diffuse skin manifestations). It can affect kidneys (renal failure), esophagus (GERD), heart (palpitations, arrhythmia), lungs (interstitial lung disease, pulmonary hypertension), and musculoskeletal (symmetrical joint pain).

Diagnosis: antinuclear antibodies (sensitive, but not specific), anti-topoisomerase antibody is more specific but present only in less than 50% of cases.

Treat symptomatically

Tumor	Features
Hemangioblastoma	• Associated with Von-Hippel Lindau syndrome ('vhl gene' mutation on chromosome 3) • Multiple tumors in cerebellum, brain stem, spinal cord and retina
Hemangioma 	Benign condition in an infant. It can occur on skin, mucous membranes or internal organs. Broadly classified into: • Capillary (strawberry and cherry hemangioma) • Cavernous **Capillary:** facial lesions in newborns, grows rapidly after birth and regresses with age **(strawberry hemangioma)** Hemangioma in elders do not regress with age, always cutaneous location (not mucosal) **(cherry hemangioma)** **Cavernous:** benign tumor of liver and spleen, rupture can complicate into hypotensive shock and hemoperitoneum.
Glomus tumor	• Benign small painful tumor of glomus body that occurs usually under fingernails from arteriovenous shunts in glomus body. • Glomus body's primary function is thermoregulation.
Angiomyolipoma 	• It is a benign tumor of kidney that is composed of blood vessels, muscle cells, and adipose tissue. • If the dilated vessels in angiomyolipoma ruptures, it will cause retroperitoneal hemorrhage • If the size is > 4cm, preventive embolization is indicated, small size tumors are not treated. • Angiomyolipoma can be associated with tuberous sclerosis.
Angiosarcoma	• Commonly found in the liver of patients with exposure to PVC, arsenic and thorotrast.

- High mortality, very aggressive tumor and difficult to resect due to delay in diagnosis.

- Can occur in skin, breast, and soft tissues,

Kaposi Sarcoma

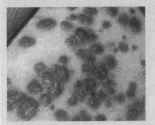

- Malignant tumor of endothelial cells.
- Associated with human herpes virus 8.
- Multiple purple patches, plaques, or nodules on skin and GI tract.
- On histology, proliferations like vascular spaces and extravasated erythrocytes can be present.

3 forms of Kaposi sarcoma are:

- **Eastern European form:** tumor is localized to skin, treat by surgical removal
- **Transplant-associated form:** treat by reducing immunosuppression
- **HIV-associated form:** highly responsive to antiretroviral therapy and interferon alpha

Bacillary Angiomatosis

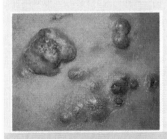

- Looks like Kaposi sarcoma. It is a benign capillary lesion in AIDS patient.

- It is caused by Bartonella hensalae. Oral erythromycin remains the drug of choice for B. hensalae.

Lymphangiosarcoma

- It is a rare lymphatic malignancy associated with persistent irritation due to lymphedema. Suspect lymphangiosarcoma in patient who develops purplish rash and ulcer on upper extremity several years after post-radical mastectomy.

Table 4.7: vascular tumors

VENOUS SYSTEM OF LEG

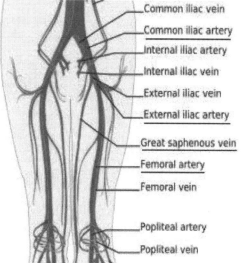

Greater and lesser saphenous veins (superficial veins) joins with a femoral vein (deep vein) at the saphenofemoral junction that forms an external iliac vein.

The external iliac vein will drain into a common iliac vein and then to inferior vena cava. Generally, the blood flows from superficial veins to deep vein.

As deep veins have higher pressure than superficial, valves present in veins prevent reversal of blood flow.

Figure 5.1: anatomy of venous system of legs*

VARICOSE VEINS

PATHOGENESIS

- The vein is dilated and tortuous (twisted) due to valve incompetence that results in reversal of blood flow from the deep veins to the superficial vein.
- It can also occur due to any obstruction in a venous system such as deep venous thrombosis. Reversal of flow will generate high pressure backward resulting in dilation of the veins.

RISK FACTORS

- Female gender
- Family history
- Multiple pregnancies
- Jobs with prolonged standing
- Obesity
- Elderly population

LOCATION

- Most common site is a superficial saphenous vein. However, it can be present in any venous system.

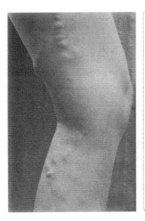 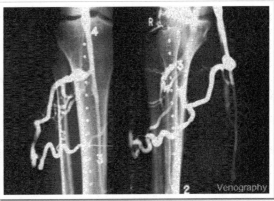

Figure 5.2: large visible varicose vein. **Figure 5.3:** tortuous (twisted) vein

CLINICAL PRESENTATION

- Skin thickening (lipodermatosclerosis)
- Large visible tortuous vein that can be visible just underneath the skin
- Ulceration
- Ache, heavy legs and ankle swelling (often worse at night and after exercise)
- Telangiectasia

COMPLICATION

Most varicose veins are benign, but severe varicosities can lead to major complications due to the poor circulation through the affected limb.

- Inability to walk

- Stasis dermatitis and venous ulcers especially near the ankle

- Severe bleeding from minor trauma

- Superficial thrombophlebitis (more serious problem if extended into deep veins)

- Acute fat necrosis

INVESTIGATION

- Confirm by duplex ultrasound, venography

MANAGEMENT

Compression hosiery is not the best but **is the best initial management**. It can help temporarily by keeping the veins empty. It includes support stocking, Ace bandages, or Unna boot. Varicose veins are treated with interventional therapy such as:

- Endothermic ablation and endovenous laser treatment of greater saphenous vein.

- If endothermal ablation is unsuitable, offer ultrasound guided foam sclerotherapy (medicine is injected, which makes varicose vein shrink).

- If foam sclerotherapy is unsuitable, offer surgery: **ligation and stripping** (removal of the vein is not a major problem because superficial vein drains only about 10% of the blood from the legs). Consider treating incompetent varicose tributaries at the same time.

THUNDERNOTE: PORTAL HYPERTENSION

- Portal hypertension is a high pressure in the hepatic portal venous system.

Cause

- Pre-hepatic (portal vein thrombosis, congenital atresia)
- Intra-hepatic (liver cirrhosis, fibrosis)
- Post-hepatic (due to cardiac problems like right heart failure, constrictive pericarditis)

Clinical Presentation

- Ascites
- Anorexia, fatigue, nausea, vomiting
- Hepatic encephalopathy
- Splenomegaly
- Gastric varicosities (dilated sub mucosal veins in stomach) and esophageal varicosities (dilated submucosal veins in lower 1/3rd esophagus). Both have high tendency to bleed, diagnosis by endoscopy.
- Anorectal varicosities (not to be confused with hemorrhoids which are due to prolapse in venous plexus of rectum) and caput medusa (which is present at the level of umbilicus)

DEEP VENOUS THROMBOSIS

Deep venous thrombosis is a blood clot in the deep veins of the leg.

- When a blood clot breaks loose and travels in the blood, this is called a venous thromboembolism. Thromboembolism from the deep veins is the most common cause (70% cases) of pulmonary embolism.
- 80% of micro pulmonary embolisms are asymptomatic due to the dual blood supply to the lung, however if the embolus is large and occludes large artery near the bifurcation of the pulmonary artery, then it can be life-threatening.

ETIOLOGY

- Venous stasis can be seen in prolonged immobilization, sedentary job (e.g. long distance truck driver), postop-patient, elders, and orthopedic casts.
- Hypercoagubility can be seen with use oral contraceptives, polycythemia vera, pancreatic cancer, antithrombin III deficiency, factor V Leiden, dysfibrinogenemia, warfarin in protein C and S deficiency.

PATHOGENESIS

- RBCs and fibrin are the main components of venous thrombi. Venous stasis and hypercoagubility are the main predisposing factors.
- Unlike atherosclerosis, venous thrombi appears attached to fibrins on a **non-thrombogenic venous endothelium**. Platelets constitute less of venous thrombi when compared to arterial ones.
- Factors like **H**ypoxia **I**nduced **F**actor and NF-κB affects thrombin production, which leads to fibrin deposition.

CLINICAL PRESENTATION

- Venous thrombosis is often asymptomatic, and can present with the 1st sign of pulmonary embolism (difficulty in breathing).
- Swelling in the affected leg (swelling is present in both legs in CHF).
- Positive Homan's sign (pain on dorsiflexion of the foot).
- Edema is due to the increase in transudate because of increase in hydrostatic pressure in distal veins.
- Stasis dermatitis, ulcers or delayed wound healing in the foot can occur due hypoxia. Stasis of blood will cause more oxygen extraction by the tissue resulting in depletion of vascular oxygen content).

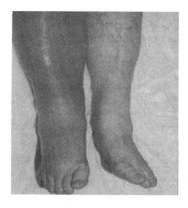 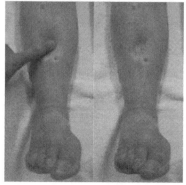

Figure 5.4: swelling in affected leg. **Figure 5.5:** pitting edema due to CHF (bilateral)

DIAGNOSIS

- Physical exam is worthless
- Venous duplex ultrasonography is the investigation of choice

MANAGEMENT

- Treat as an outpatient, if feasible.
- **In an acute setting,** i.e. the first few days; management is **with low molecular weight heparin**. The aim is to maintain PTT 2-3 times normal i.e. 50-75 seconds.
- Preferred treatment beyond the first few days: **warfarin (for 3-6 months).** INR is maintained at 2-3. Withdraw heparin once patient gets stable on warfarin.
- If the patient comes back after 10-20 days of starting warfarin with bleeding (gastrointestinal or cerebral), stop giving warfarin and place inferior vena cava filter.
- Control the primary cause responsible for venous stasis or hypercoagubility.

For mild or moderate symptoms of DVTs and no risk factors for clot extension:

- No anticoagulation needed. The physician need to obtain several Doppler ultrasound of legs over the next 2 weeks to make sure that DVT has not extended.
- If an extension of clot has not occurred within the first 2 weeks, it is unlikely to occur subsequently.

Risk factors for clot extension

- Positive D-dimer test (< 250 mg/ml = low risk of recurrence, >250 mg/ml = high risk of recurrence).

If DVT has extended

- Treat with warfarin for 3-6 months.
- For the deep venous thrombosis or pulmonary embolism associated with malignancy: Low molecular weight heparin is the preferred over warfarin.

SUPERFICIAL THROMBOPHLEBITIS

Superficial thrombophlebitis is thrombosis and inflammation of superficial veins that presents as a painful induration with erythema, often in a linear or branching configuration; forming cords. Thrombophlebitis can develop along the arm, back, or neck veins; the leg (saphenous veins) is by far the most common site.

ETIOLOGY

- Prolonged catheterization of veins
- Infections (most commonly by S. aureus)
- Visceral malignancies like pancreatic cancer (trousseau sign: migratory superficial thrombophlebitis)
- Hypercoagulable states and other causes of deep venous thrombosis.

CLINICAL PRESENTATION

- Thrombophlebitis is a self-limited disorder that often presents with tenderness, induration, pain and/or erythema along the course of a superficial vein
- Palpable nodular cord can be felt due to the thrombus within the affected vein. Persistence of this cord when the extremity is raised suggests the presence of thrombus

COMPLICATION

- Deep vein thrombosis, varicose veins and ulcers in foot

DIAGNOSIS

- Clinical presentation and Duplex ultrasound

MANAGEMENT

- Compression stockings (warm, moist compressions with Unna boot), NSAIDs

- Anticoagulants (if involved vein segment is > 5 cm and proximal to saphenofemoral junction)

- If everything fails, perform surgery

LEG ULCERS			
Diabetic	**Arterial Insufficiency**	**Venous Stasis**	**Malignancy**
Located at pressure point (heel, metatarsal head, tip of toes)	Located at area with low blood flow (tip of toes)	Located anywhere in chronically edematous and indurated skin (usually above the medial malleolus)	Located anywhere depending upon the chronic injury
The neuropathy and microvascular disease plays important role in development of ulcer. A person is usually unaware of developing ulcer (because no nerve sensations).	Primary mechanism of ulcer is ischemia - In arterial insufficiency – decreased delivery of oxygen. Less blood volume. - In venous stasis – oxygen is used up from the stagnant blood (low oxygen saturation). High blood volume.		Due to previously untreated ulcer for long period (e.g. 3rd-degree burn that underwent spontaneous healing, chronic draining sinuses due to osteomyelitis)

Advise the patient to check their feet daily once diagnosed with diabetic neuropathy (preventive measures).	Signs of peripheral artery disease will be present. Dirty looking ulcer with pale base devoid of granulation tissue.	Painless ulcer with granulation tissue base. The patient may have a history of varicose vein and history of cellulitis.	Dirty looking deep ulcer with heaped up tissue at the edge Biopsy is diagnostic Surgery is best (wide excision)

DIAGNOSIS

- Look for the other clinical manifestations.
- Doppler studies to differentiate the primary cause of the ulcer.
- Calculate the ABI ratio (ankle-brachial pressure ratio). A **value of 0.5 or less is unlikely to be venous pathology**, 0.6 to 0.9 is peripheral artery disease or mixed arterial-venous, and **value greater than 0.9 excludes arterial pathology.**
- Angiography is most accurate for peripheral artery disease.
- Diabetic and atherosclerosis-related ulcers usually coexist together and thus all patients with chronic ulcer must be evaluated for diabetes and atherosclerosis.
- Chronic or recurrent ulcers must be biopsied to exclude malignancy

MANAGEMENTS

- None of them will heal on its own unless the primary cause is managed.
- Treat the primary cause as soon as possible because the next stage is dry gangrene and once bacteria will superimpose the ulcer, it will convert to wet gangrene and patient might require amputation. Prevention is the best way and all patients with diabetes and peripheral arterial disease must be guided for this.
- For ulcers due to arterial insufficiency, managements are similar to the peripheral arterial disease. Surgical revascularization might be required.
- For ulcers due to venous stasis, primary management is supportive with stockings, bandages, and Unna boot (replace every 10 days). If primary managements fail, do surgery or endovascular ablation.
- For ulcers due to malignancy, surgical excision must be performed.

Table 5.1: leg ulcers

EVALUATION OF CHEST PAIN

Any elderly patient who presents with anginal chest pain (dull, squeezing substernal chest pain) must be evaluated for acute coronary syndrome.

If the patient is hemodynamically stable, obtain focused history, assess vital signs and perform chest x-ray and ECG. Administer aspirin if the risk of aortic dissection is low.

- If ECG is consistent with ST-elevated myocardial infarction, best initial step in management is emergency thrombolysis or PCI unless contraindicated.
- If ECG is consistent with non-ST-elevated myocardial infarction, best initial step in management is low molecular weight heparin.

If the ECG findings are inconsistent with acute coronary syndrome, check chest x-ray, cardiac markers and risk stratify for acute coronary syndrome. Assess for pulmonary embolism, pericarditis, aortic dissection and treat appropriately. Details are discussed in subsequent chapters.

The most common cause of chest pain in elderly population is gastroesophageal reflux disease. If the cardiac markers are normal and risk for acute coronary syndrome is low, suspect gastroesophageal reflux disease.

ISCHEMIC HEART DISEASE

- Ischemic heart disease is due to an imbalance between myocardial oxygen demand and supply from the coronary arteries.
- Coronary artery disease is the number one cause of death in the United States. Ischemia occurs secondary to the coronary artery disease.
- Atherosclerosis is the number one cause of coronary artery disease.
- Hypertension is the number one cause for atherosclerosis while diabetes and smoking are the most dangerous causes for coronary artery disease.

STABLE ANGINA

- Main cause: atherosclerotic occlusion of the coronary arteries (>70%).

- The appearance of anginal chest pain occurs during exertions like exercise, climbing staircase or emotional stress.

- Patient often complains of sub-sternal chest tightness-heaviness and dull-sore-squeezing sub-sternal pain that may radiates to the neck or left arm (because the sympathetic fibers from T1-T2 will supply both the heart and left arm, jaw).

- Pain disappears by rest or sublingual nitroglycerine.

UNSTABLE ANGINA

- Unstable angina is also called as acute coronary syndrome. It will have all symptoms of anginal chest pain **at rest.**

- Chest discomfort does not improve with nitroglycerine or recurs soon after nitroglycerine.

- The lumen of the coronary artery is not completely occluded by the thrombus. It has a high risk for myocardial infarction. Irreversible changes in cardiac myocytes begins after 20-25 minutes of ischemia.

PRINZMETAL ANGINA

- Chest pain occurs due to the episodes of coronary artery vasospasm. Atherosclerotic narrowing of lumen is not present.

- A possible mechanism behind this is an increase in platelet thromboxane A2 and endothelin (a potent vasoconstrictor).

- Prinzmetal angina produces chest pain at rest; more commonly in the morning on waking up.

- Unlike unstable angina, Prinzmetal angina will be relieved by nitroglycerine.

- Calcium channel blockers are preferred over the beta-blockers in the management.

- During the episodes, transmural ischemia will occur that will cause ST-segment elevation on ECG.

MYOCARDIAL INFARCTION

- Myocardial infarction will present similarly to unstable angina. It is not possible to distinguish between them solely base on clinical presentation. Positive cardiac enzyme test is indicative of MI.

- Lumen of the coronary artery is completely occluded due atherosclerotic plaque rupture and superimposed thrombus formation or coronary artery spasm.

- Serum cardiac markers will be released into the blood due to cell lysis/death. Cardiac markers will not be present in blood if cardiac myocyte is not dead.

RISK FACTOR

- Age (male > 55 years, female > 65 years) is the most important risk factor. There is less than 2% chance of having MI in a young woman at age 25 compared to 65-year-old female.

- Family history: multiple gene inheritances.

- Lipid abnormalities: leads to atherosclerosis; LDL > 160 mg/dl, HDL < 40 mg/dl.

- Environmental: smoking, lifestyle, drugs (cocaine); hypertension and diabetes.

- Previous myocardial infarction

- Congestive heart failure, mitral valve dysfunction, aortic dissection, aortic aneurysm

- Atrial or ventricular arrhythmia

- Hypercoagulable states (polycythemia, antithrombin III deficiency)

- Vasculitis (polyarteritis nodosa, Kawasaki disease)

DIFFERENTIAL DIAGNOSIS

- Gastroesophageal reflux disease and peptic ulcer disease is the most common cause of epigastric pain. Pain is related to certain food, and relieved by antacids.

- Stable angina (pain on exertion, ST segment depression)

- Unstable angina (pain at rest, ST segment depression)

- Diffuse esophageal spasms (normal ECG, abnormal gastrointestinal series)

- Pericarditis (diffuse ST-segment elevation, PR depression, pain relieved on leaning forward)

- Pulmonary embolism (pleuritic chest pain, prolonged immobilization)

- Costochondritis (tenderness on palpation)

- Aortic dissection (pain radiating to the back, widened mediastinum)

- Tension pneumothorax (absent breath sound on affected side, often post-trauma)

- Prinzmetal angina (pain at rest, ST elevation during episodes)

POST MI COMPLICATIONS

- Cardiac arrest: most commonly occurs due to the ventricular fibrillation and is the most common cause of death following an MI.

- Bradyarrhythmia: atrioventricular block is more common following inferior wall MI.

- Pericarditis: acute pericarditis in the first 48 hours following a transmural MI is common (10% cases).

- Left ventricular free wall rupture: this is seen in around 3% cases of MI and occurs after 5-7 days. The patient will present with acute heart failure secondary to cardiac tamponade (raised JVP, pulsus paradoxus, diminished heart sounds). Urgent pericardiocentesis and thoracotomy are required.

- Ventricular septal defect: rupture of the interventricular septum usually occurs in the first week and is seen in around 1-2% of patients. An echocardiogram is diagnostic and will exclude acute mitral regurgitation, which presents in a similar fashion. Urgent surgical correction is needed.

- Acute mitral regurgitation: more common with posterior wall infarction and occurs due to the rupture of the papillary muscle. An early-to-mid systolic murmur is typically heard. Emergency surgical repair is required. Anything that has an acute presentation in the heart carries bad prognosis and must be treated emergently.

- Cardiogenic shock: if a large part of the ventricular myocardium is damaged in the infarction, ejection fraction of the heart may decrease to the point that the patient develops cardiogenic shock. Other causes of cardiogenic shock include 'mechanical' complications such as left ventricular free wall rupture.

- Congestive heart failure: If the patient survives the acute phase their ventricular myocardium may be dysfunctional resulting in chronic heart failure.

- Left ventricular aneurysm: the ischemic damage sustained may weaken the myocardium resulting in aneurysm formation. This is typically associated with persistent ST elevation and left ventricular failure. The thrombus may form within an aneurysm increasing the risk of stroke.

- **DRESSLER SYNDROME:** It is an immune-mediated pericarditis that can occur several weeks after an MI.

  Pathogenesis: the underlying pathophysiology is thought to be an autoimmune reaction against the antigenic proteins on the myocardium.

Clinical presentation: the patient often describes the pain that is worse with deep inspiration and improves on leaning forward.

Diagnosis: clinical presentation and ECG findings of normal QRS complex, ST-segment elevation and PR-depression in all leads (reciprocal in lead V1).

Management: the best initial management of Dressler's syndrome is NSAIDs.

Time	Microscopic Change	Gross Change	Complications
1-4 hours	No change	No change	Cardiogenic shock, congestive heart failure, arrhythmia
24-hours	Coagulative necrosis (removal of nucleus; pyknosis, karyorrhexis, karyolysis)	Dark discoloration	Arrhythmia (due to damage in conductive pathway), If no arrhythmia within 24 hours of MI, 90% less probability of having one later.
1-3 days	Numerous neutrophils (due to acute inflammation following necrosis)	Yellow discoloration	Fibrinous pericarditis (transmural infarctions)
3-7 days	Numerous macrophages (will clean up the necrotic debris). The infarcted wall is weakest around this time.	Yellow pallor	Ventricular free wall rupture (leads to cardiac tamponade), interventricular septum rupture (left to right shunt), Papillary muscles rupture (mitral insufficiency)
2 weeks	Granulation tissue with fibroblast, collagen and blood vessels (reconstruction of infarcted wall)	Central pallor with red border	-
1 Month	Fibrosis (scar formation)	White discoloration	Aneurysm, Dressler syndrome

Table 6.1: Post-MI changes

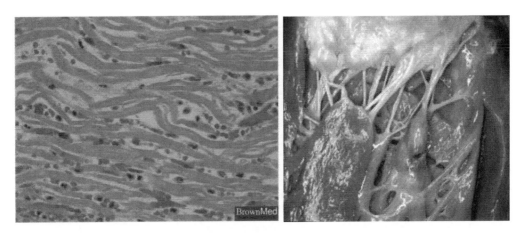

Figure 6.1: wavy fibers (1-4 hours) *, **Figure 6.2:** papillary muscle rupture (1-week) *

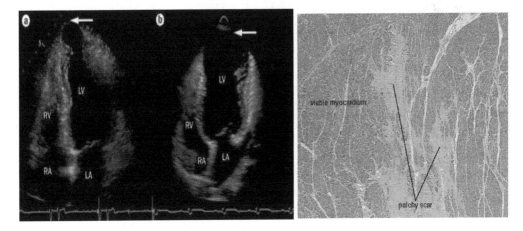

Figure 6.3: left ventricular aneurysm (1-month) *, **Figure 6.4:** scar tissue (1-month) *

Post-MI ECG Changes in STEMI

- Unstable angina (before the actual MI): T wave inversion

- **Within hours after MI: marked ST-segment elevation + upright T wave**

- After 24 hours: Significant Q wave + ST-segment elevation + upright T wave

- After 48 hours: Significant Q wave + less ST-segment elevation + inverted T wave

- After 1-2 weeks: Significant Q wave + No ST-segment elevation + inverted T wave

- **After 1-2 months: Significant Q wave only**

ST-SEGMENT ELEVATION

ST elevation >1mm in the limb leads and >2mm in the chest lead indicates an evolving acute MI until there is proof to the contrary. ST-segment elevation can also be present in:

- Early ventricular repolarization (normal variant in young adults)
- Pericarditis
- Ventricular aneurysm
- Pulmonary embolism
- Intracranial hemorrhage

ST-SEGMENT DEPRESSION

Non-ST-segment elevated MI (NSTEMI) are difficult to distinguish from unstable angina on ECG. Cardiac markers are elevated in NSTEMI while cardiac markers are normal in unstable angina. ST-segment depression can be present in:

- Myocardial ischemia
- Unstable angina
- Left ventricular hypertrophy
- Intraventricular conduction defects
- Medications (digitalis)
- Reciprocal changes in leads opposite to the area of acute injury (lead V1)

12-LEAD ECG INTERPRETATIONS

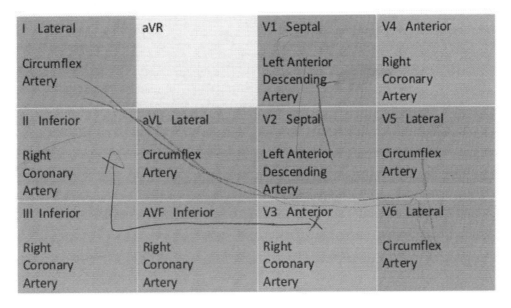

I Lateral	aVR	V1 Septal	V4 Anterior
Circumflex Artery		Left Anterior Descending Artery	Right Coronary Artery
II Inferior	aVL Lateral	V2 Septal	V5 Lateral
Right Coronary Artery	Circumflex Artery	Left Anterior Descending Artery	Circumflex Artery
III Inferior	AVF Inferior	V3 Anterior	V6 Lateral
Right Coronary Artery	Right Coronary Artery	Right Coronary Artery	Circumflex Artery

Figure 6.5: coronary arteries and 12-leads*

- **Left circumflex artery** supply blood to lateral wall of left ventricle, left atrium and left posterior fasciculus of left bundle branch. Occlusion will cause lateral wall MI. Reciprocal ST depression in inferior leads (III and vVF).

- **Left anterior descending** artery supply blood to anterior wall of left ventricle, anterior 2/3rd interventricular septum, bundle of his, right bundle branch and left anterior fasciculus of left bundle branch. Occlusion will cause septal MI.

- **Right coronary artery** supply blood to right atrium, right ventricles, posterior and inferior wall of left ventricle. Occlusion will cause inferior wall MI (commonly seen together with posterior wall MI)

I A L

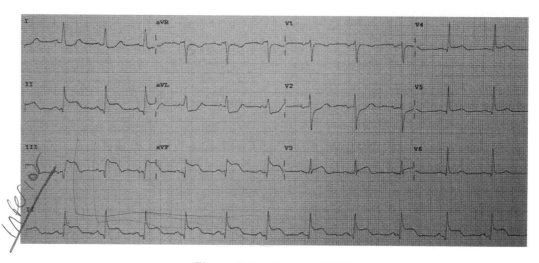

Figure 6.6: inferior wall MI*

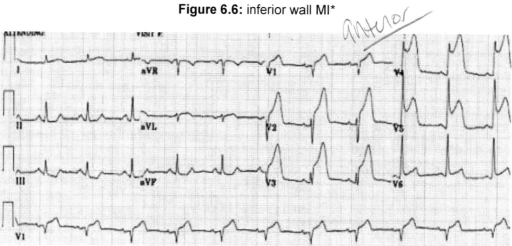

anterior

Figure 6.7: anterior wall MI*

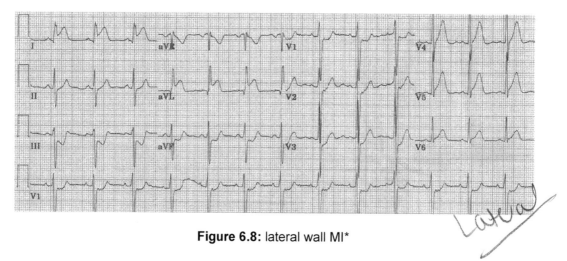

Lateral

Figure 6.8: lateral wall MI*

PHYSICAL EXAMINATION

- Normal in the absence of an anginal attack.

- MI is diagnosed if the anginal attacks occur more than 20 minutes.

- Look for heart failure signs (shortness of breath, increased JVP, bibasilar crackles, edema in legs) from prior MI.

- Rule out other possible causes of chest pain such as costochondritis, pericarditis.

PRETEST PROBABILITY OF CORONARY ARTERY DISEASE

- <10 % probability in asymptomatic patient and woman less than 50 years with atypical angina: **do nothing.**

- 10-90% probability in men with atypical chest pain and age more than 50 years: **do stress test if ECG is normal.**

- >90% probability in woman greater than 60 years with typical chest pain (angina-like) or a man older than 40 years with typical angina: **If ECG is normal, go directly to angiography.**

DIAGNOSIS

- Best first step in patient's with moderate to severe probability of having acute coronary syndrome is always an ECG.

- If ECG is inconclusive (NSTEMI can have ST depression or normal), go for a exercise stress test or thallium echo (don't give dipyridamole in patients with reactive lung disease and it is generally not preferred when exercise stress test is a possible alternative). Both tests are equivalent.

- If ECG test shows STEMI or for individuals with high probability, a coronary angiogram can be used to definitively diagnose or rule out coronary artery disease.

- Coronary angiography should be performed **after stabilizing a patient** with medical therapy, but emergency angiography may be undertaken in unstable patients.

- In patients with unstable angina/NSTEMI, the TIMI risk score is a simple prognostication scheme that categorizes a patient's risk of death and ischemic events and provides a basis for therapeutic decision-making.

- For prinzmetal angina, ST elevation on ECG is not specific. Angiography is done to exclude possible acute coronary syndrome. Prinzmetal angina can be suspected when angiogram is normal.

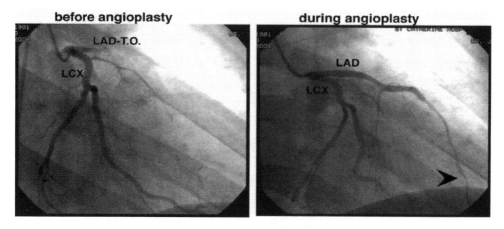

Figure 6.9: Coronary angiogram showing a total occlusion of left anterior descending artery and a normal left circumflex coronary artery (LCX). Angioplasty restored flow with distal filling defects due to a residual thrombus*

THUNDERNOTE: TIMI SCORE

The TIMI score predicts the risk of all-cause mortality, MI and severe recurrent ischemia requiring urgent revascularization within 14 days after admission as well as the benefit of enoxaparin.

TIMI Score Calculation (1 point for each): Mnemonic - AMERICA

- Age greater than 65
- Markers: Elevated serum cardiac biomarkers
- ECG: ST changes of at least 0.5mm on admission ECG
- Risk factors: at least 3 risk factors for coronary artery disease, such as;
    1. Hypertension > 140/90 or on antihypertensive drugs
    2. Current cigarette smoker
    3. Low HDL cholesterol (< 40 mg/dL) or high LDL > 160mg/dL
    4. Diabetes mellitus
    5. The family history of premature coronary artery disease (coronary artery disease in male first-degree relative, or father less than 55, or female first-degree relative or mother less than 65).
- Ischemia: at-least 2 anginal episodes within last 24hrs
- Coronary artery disease: Coronary stenosis greater than 50%

- Aspirin use in the last 7 days (patient experiences chest pain despite aspirin used in past 7 days)

SCORE:

0-1= Low risk

2-3 = Intermediate risk

4 or above = High risk

High HDL > 40mg/dL subtracts 1 point.

Cardiac Markers:

- Myoglobin: it is detected from 1 to 5 hour of chest pain.

  Normal myoglobin means no MI, however if myoglobin is elevated, it is non-specific; It can be MI or something else. No Troponins or CK-MB will be detected until 4-7 hours of an onset of acute MI..

- Troponin I will start rising by 4th hour, peaks at 16 hours and remain elevated for 7-10 days (usually drawn every 8 hours three times till MI is ruled out)

- Creatinine Kinase-MB will start rising by 4th hour, peaks at 20 hours and disappears on the 3rd day of an acute MI. It is used to detect re-infarction because troponin level will be high for 10 days.

- CK-MB have sensitivity and specificity of 95%. Troponin I is more specific than CK-MB because CK-MB can also be elevated in rhabdomyolysis, myocarditis or other conditions (differentiated based on clinical presentation).

  Troponin I along with CK-MB improves overall sensitivity and specificity for MI.

MANAGEMENT

- Any patient with moderate-severe probability of acute coronary syndrome, who complains about pain typical for angina, give aspirin and nitroglycerine (given sublingually or by spray) as soon as possible even before performing an ECG or placing IV access line.

ACUTE MANAGEMENT FOR STEMI

- The decision must be made quickly as to whether the patient should be treated with thrombolysis or with primary percutaneous coronary intervention (PCI).

  PCI is superior to thrombolytic (mortality benefits, less chance of developing post-MI complications, fewer complications like hemorrhage).

- In the absence of contraindications, give thrombolytic (tissue plasminogen activator) within 12 hours of anginal attack. Ideally, thrombolytic medications should be given within first 30 minutes of patient's arrival at the hospital. After thrombolytic therapy, patient must be transferred for angiography.

- If pain persists after initial thrombolytic therapy, schedule the patient for PCI.

- GP IIb/IIIa inhibitors such as abciximab or eptifibatide or tirofiban is added to aspirin after PCI to prevent a clot.

- Placement of stents coated with sirolimus/paclitaxel decreases the risk of restenosis (by 90%) as compared to bare metal stents (75-80%). Clopidogrel is given for 1-year in patients with stents coated with sirolimus/paclitaxel and for 1-month for bare metal stents.

ACUTE MANAGEMENT FOR NSTEMI

- NSTEMI patients are not a candidate for immediate thrombolytic. Thrombolytics such as streptokinase, and tissue plasminogen activator are not helpful in NSTEMI and is not preferred.

- They should receive anti-ischemic therapy; **low molecular weight heparin** and if pain persists then may be candidates for PCI urgently or during admission.

THUNDERNOTE: CONTRAINDICATIONS FOR THROMBOLYTICS

Absolute contraindication

- History of intracranial hemorrhage
- Ischemic stroke within 3 months
- Cerebral structural lesions
- Malignant intracranial neoplasm
- Intracranial surgery within 2 months
- Active bleeding or bleeding diathesis (except menses)
- Uncontrolled hypertensive emergency

Relative contraindications (give thrombolytic if benefits outweigh the risk and PCI is not available):

- Hypertensive crisis
- Major surgery less than 3 weeks previously
- History of Ischemic stroke before 3 months
- Recent internal bleeding within 4 weeks
- Pregnancy
- Current warfarin use

INDICATIONS FOR PCI and CABG

- PCI like angioplasty is indicated if 1 coronary vessel is occluded other than the main left coronary artery.

- CABG is more effective when 2 vessels with serious risk factors such as diabetes, 3 vessels or left main coronary artery are occluded (saphenous vein, Internal thoracic artery are frequently used).

- In 2 or 3 vessel disease, if right coronary artery (inferior wall MI) is involved, we first do stenting emergently in right coronary artery and then schedule the patient for CABG. CABG is rarely done in an emergency. When harvesting is done, the patient is given heparin to prevent the blood from clotting.

LONG TERM MANAGEMENT

- All patients with acute MI should receive aspirin and prasugrel (better choice than clopidogrel) in the absence of any contraindication.

  In patients with aspirin allergy: use clopidogrel

  If both aspirin and clopidogrel fails: use ticlopidine.

- High-intensity statin therapy is given to everybody. The goal is to maintain LDL level less than 100mg/dL.

- Sublingual nitroglycerin to is given to abort angina attacks. Advise the patient; when and how to take it.

- Beta-blockers are generally used as a first-line rhythm control drug for chronic management.

- Calcium channel blocker like verapamil is used when beta blockers are contraindicated (asthma with wheezing and 2nd degree AV block). Selective beta-blockers like metoprolol are not contraindicated for a patient with the previous history of COPD with no wheezing or difficulty in breathing at the time of presentation. Increase the dose in case of poor drug response [do not stop the drug abruptly because beta-adrenergic receptors are super-sensitized with long term beta blocker therapy].

- If a calcium channel blocker is used as monotherapy, verapamil or diltiazem should be used. If used in combination with a beta-blocker, then use a long-acting dihydropyridine calcium-channel blocker such as nifedipine. Remember that beta-blockers should not be prescribed concurrently with verapamil.

- If a patient is on monotherapy and cannot tolerate the addition of a calcium channel blocker or a beta-blocker then consider one of the following drugs: a long-acting nitrate, ivabradine, nicorandil, or ranolazine.

- If a patient is taking both a beta-blocker and a calcium channel blocker (dihydropyridine group) then add third drug only when a patient is awaiting assessment for PCI or CABG.

- ACE inhibitors are indicated for all acute MI. They are most effective when ejection fraction is less than 40%. If the patient develops chronic cough on ACE inhibitor, switch it to angiotensin receptor blocker (ARBs).

- Furosemide work favorably and do not interfere with the effects of ACE inhibitors. It is indicated for all patient with high blood pressure and volume overload in failing heart.

POST MI PRECAUTIONS

- Do stress test after 5 days or prior to discharging patient. If the test is positive: recommend not to involve in any sexual activity for 2-6 weeks. Male on the bottom and female on the top is better position in heart failure patients. If the test is negative: he can have sex whenever he wants.

- Do not give nitrates with sildenafil due to the risk of severe hypotension.

- Both beta-blockers and anxiety can cause sexual dysfunction post-MI. Reassure the patient and help him to cope with anxiety.

- Lifestyle change such as weight loss, smoking cessation, low salt diet, aerobic exercise, and healthy diet is recommended.

THUNDERNOTE: INDICATIONS FOR STATIN

Four statin benefit groups which demonstrated a maximum reduction in outcomes associated with atherosclerotic cardiovascular disease (ASCVD) are:

1) Individuals with clinical ASCVD (acute coronary syndromes, history of myocardial infarction, stable or unstable angina, stroke or peripheral arterial disease presumed to be of atherosclerotic origin)

2) Individuals with LDL cholesterol ≥190 mg/dl.

3) Individuals 40-75 years of age with diabetes and LDL cholesterol 100-189 mg/dl without clinical ASCVD.

4) Individuals without clinical ASCVD or diabetes, who are 40-75 years of age with LDL-C 70-189 mg/dl and have an estimated 10-year ASCVD risk of 7.5% or higher (**Age >75** without any other risk factors, alone have 10-year ASCVD risk >7.5%)

In selected individuals who does not fall in above 4 categories, whether to initiate statin therapy or not is still unclear. Additional risk factors must be considered.

Recommendations for High-intensity statin therapy:

- All patients with **age less than 75 years** and have MI, stable/unstable angina, stroke, transient ischemic attack, peripheral arterial disease
- All patients with diabetics with 10-year ASCVD risk >7.5%
- LDL >190mg/dL at any time

Recommendations for Moderate intensity statin therapy:

- All patients with **age more than 75 years** and have acute coronary syndrome, MI, stable/unstable angina, stroke, transient ischemic attack, peripheral arterial disease
- Diabetics with 10-year ASCVD risk <7.5%
- Estimated 10-year risk of ASCVD in non-diabetics >7.5%

High-intensity statin therapy is defined as a daily dose that lowers LDL-C by ≥50% and moderate-intensity statin therapy lowers LDL-C by 30%.

Lifestyle modification (healthy diet, regular exercise, avoidance of tobacco products, and maintenance of a healthy weight) remains a critical component of health promotion and ASCVD risk reduction***.

- High-intensity statins dose: Rosuvastatin 20-40mg daily, Atorvastatin 40-80mg daily

- Moderate-intensity statins dose: Atorvastatin 10-20mg daily, Rosuvastatin 5-10mg daily, Simvastatin 20-40mg daily, Pravastatin 40-80mg daily, Lovastatin 40mg daily.

[** Dosages are not tested on USMLE but it is important to remember indications for high-intensity and low-intensity statin therapy for Step 3]

REPERFUSION INJURY

- Reperfusion injury is the tissue damage that occurs when the blood supply returns to the tissue after a period of ischemia or lack of oxygen. It can be observed after thrombolysis for acute-MI, PCI, and CABG.

- The absence of oxygen and nutrients from blood during the ischemic period creates a condition in which the restoration of circulation results in inflammation and oxidative damage through the induction of oxidative stress rather than restoration of normal function.

- Reperfusion injury can cause myocardial stunning, microvascular dysfunction (vasoconstriction; no-reflow after reperfusion therapy) and even death. Histological section will show myofibril thinning and wavy pattern.

- Although, inotropic stimulation is not an ideal strategy to counter reperfusion injury, it is effective and not associated with worsening of injury. Transient inotropic support is routinely used for a stunned re-perfused myocardium in variety of settings, however, there is no definitive therapy.

THUNDERNOTE: Myocardial Stunning and Hibernation

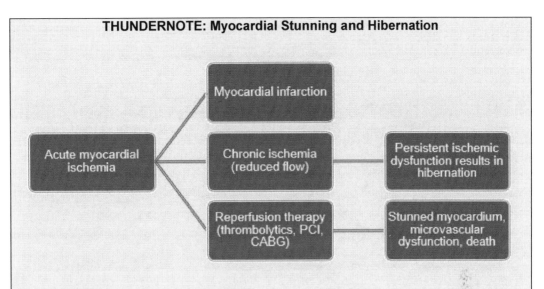

Myocardial Stunning

- When ischemia is severe and prolonged, it causes myocyte death and results in loss of contractile function and tissue infarction.
- In cases of less severe ischemia, some myocytes remain viable but have depressed contractile function. This phenomenon of prolonged depression of regional function **after a reversible episode of ischemia** is called as myocardial stunning
- Normally myocardium will regain full function in 5 minutes after reperfusion, however, stunned myocardium will take hours to recover.

2 major hypotheses for myocardial stunning:

- Oxygen-free radical hypothesis.
- Calcium overload hypothesis.

Inotropic agents like dobutamine or epinephrine will improve the contractility.

Hibernating myocardium

- A state of persistently impaired myocardial and left ventricular function at rest due to reduced coronary blood flow that can be partially or completely restored to normal either by improving blood flow or by reducing oxygen demand.

- Stunning and hibernation are believed to be an adaptive process to protect myocardium against free radical injury (stunning) or reduced coronary flow (hibernation).

Respiratory arrest	Cardiac arrest	Heart attack (MI)
No breathing due to problem in the lungs.	Heart stops beating all of a sudden; leading to ceasing of circulation. The problem is in the heart rhythm.	Sudden stop in blood supply to part of heart due to atherosclerotic plaque rupture (myocardial infarction)
Predisposing conditions: amyotrophic lateral sclerosis, cerebrovascular stroke, acute lung injury, myopathy, asthma attack and drowning	Predisposing conditions: coronary heart disease (65%), cardiomyopathy, cardiac rhythm disturbances, hypertensive heart disease, congestive heart failure, trauma, pulmonary embolus.	Atherosclerosis is the main cause for an MI. MI is the most common cause for cardiac arrest.
Respiratory arrest can be caused by or can cause cardiac arrest. Breathing stops first resulting in an inadequate cerebral and cardiac oxygen delivery. This will cause loss of consciousness and cardiac arrest.	Heart stops beating though it still receives a constant supply of oxygenated blood. Due to inadequate cerebral perfusion, the person will stop breathing and lose consciousness. It can lead neuronal damage in 3 minutes or death in 5 minutes (sudden cardiac death)	Infarcted area of the heart does not receive the oxygenated blood and all the while it continues to beat and pump blood until the cells die completely.
All conditions are medical emergency and should be managed appropriately.		

Table 6.2: concepts of cardiac arrest and respiratory arrest

The loss of consciousness due to the cardiac causes is by far more common than the loss of consciousness due to the primary pulmonary cause. ABC is now replaced by CAB with certain exceptions for newborn with airway obstruction or any drowning situation. Do CAB when primary cause is not clear. CAB is recommended at first place in person with sudden fall and loss of consciousness (by not doing airway/breathing before compression, we can save up to 20% more patients). A universal compression to ventilation ratio is of 30:2 (15:2 in children). Recommended compression depth is 5 cm in adult and children. In adults perform compression with 2 hands, in children with 1 hand and in newborns with 2 fingers.

Emergency note # 1

- Under non-clinical setting, when you see an unresponsive person who just fell on the ground; CALL 911 first or ask somebody to do so and then start compression immediately. Do not try to be super hero by first trying compressions and seeing whether a person becomes responsive and then call 911. He might require defibrillation if he has ventricular arrhythmia.

Emergency note # 2

- If AED (Automated External Defibrillator) is available and patient is unconscious/not breathing, deliver 1 shock first.

- Perform chest compressions at a rate of 100/minute. After 30 compressions clear the airway and ventilate by mouth twice. If the patient is still having ventricular fibrillation or pulseless ventricular tachycardia, then defibrillate again or continue CPR till the arrival of ambulance.

- If the heart rhythm is not restored, besides CPR and defibrillation, **add** IV epinephrine after 2nd shock.

- If the patient continues to have **ventricular arrhythmias** (ventricular fibrillation or pulseless ventricular tachycardia), **add** antiarrhythmic like procainamide or lidocaine after 3rd shock. For arrhythmias due to prolong QT interval; procainamide or amiodarone are contraindicated, **use lidocaine after 3rd shock.**

- Continue defibrillation-CPR cycle at least 4-5 times. This is the best effort that you can do to save the patient.

- During pregnancy when a woman is lying on her back, the uterus may compress the inferior vena cava and thus decrease venous return. It is therefore recommended that the uterus is pushed to the woman's left; if this is not effective, either roll the woman 30° or consider emergency caesarean section.

THUNDERNOTE: Percutaneous Coronary Interventions

- PCI include percutaneous transluminal coronary angioplasty (PTCA) with or without stent insertion.

Procedure

- PTCA is done via percutaneous femoral, radial, or brachial artery puncture.

- A guiding catheter is inserted into a large peripheral artery and threaded to the appropriate coronary ostium.

- A balloon-tipped catheter, guided by fluoroscopy or intravascular ultrasonography, is aligned within the stenosis, and then inflated to disrupt the atherosclerotic plaque and dilate the artery.

- Angiography is repeated after the procedure to document any changes. The procedure is commonly done in 2 or 3 vessels as needed.

Stents

Stents are most useful for

- Short lesions in large native coronary arteries not previously treated with PTCA

- Focal lesions in saphenous vein grafts

- Treatment of abrupt closure during PTCA

Stents are now used frequently for acute MI, ostial or left main coronary disease, chronic total occlusions, and bifurcation lesions.

Types of stents:

- Bare metal stents are made of nickel-titanium alloy.

- Drug-eluting stents are coated with sirolimus, everolimus, or zotarolimus that limits intimal proliferation and reduces the risk of restenosis.

- Radioactive stents had not proven effective at limiting restenosis. Biodegradable stents are currently in clinical trials.

Anticoagulation

- Thienopyridines (clopidogrel, prasugrel, ticagrelor) and glycoprotein IIb/IIIa inhibitors are the standard of care for patients with unstable NSTEMI. Thienopyridines in combination with aspirin are continued for 9 to 12 months after PCI. Calcium channel blockers and nitrates may also reduce the risk of coronary spasm.

Contraindication

Absolute contraindication:

- Lack of cardiac surgical support
- Critical left main coronary stenosis without collateral flow from a native vessel or **previous bypass graft** to the left anterior descending artery

Relative contraindication:

- Coagulopathy
- Diffusely diseased vessels without focal stenosis
- A single diseased vessel providing all perfusion to the myocardium
- Total occlusion of a coronary artery
- Stenosis < 50%

Complication

- One of the main complication of balloon angioplasty and stent placement is thromboses (acute: immediately, subacute: <30 days, late: >30 days).
- Restenosis (due to collagen deposition, occurs after several weeks).
- Arterial dissection
- PCI has the highest risk of contrast nephropathy; this risk can be reduced by pre-procedural hydration and possibly by use of a nonionic contrast agent or hemofiltration in patients with preexisting renal insufficiency.
- Stent placement, in addition to the above, has complications of bleeding secondary to aggressive adjunctive anticoagulation, side branch occlusion, and stent embolism.

Takotsubo cardiomyopathy is also called as broken heart syndrome or apical ballooning cardiomyopathy or stress cardiomyopathy. It is found in 1-2% cases that are presented with acute coronary syndrome. Women are more commonly affected with a mean age of 60-75 years.

Takotsubo cardiomyopathy is a nonischemic, sudden weakening of myocardium. 75% cases are associated with emotional stress like the death of loved ones, divorce etc. and thus called as broken heart syndrome. Rest 20% cases has no association or occur more in winter.

ETIOLOGY

- No specific cause has been identified yet

- There are many different theories such as; some amount of idiopathic vasospasm, microvasculature failure, myocardial stunning (catecholamine induced - most supported).

CLINICAL PRESENTATION

- Diagnosis is difficult based on the initial presentation. It mimics anterior wall myocardial infarction and therefore, most common symptom is acute substernal chest pain.

- The most common ECG finding is ST segment elevation in anterior leads with T-wave inversion and QT prolongation.

COMPLICATION

- Complications can be seen in the early course of disease such as; ventricular arrhythmia, heart failure, bradyarrhythmia, mitral regurgitation, or cardiogenic shock.

DIAGNOSIS

- Evaluate the patient just like myocardial infarction.

- On echocardiography, base of the ventricles contracts normally or hyperkinetic but the apex is not contracting (akinetic) and looks like ballooned left ventricular apex during systole (looks normal during diastole).

- Angiography will not reveal any significant stenosis in vessels and cardiac MRI will not show gadolinium enhancement (subendocardial or transmural gadolinium enhancement in seen in MI).

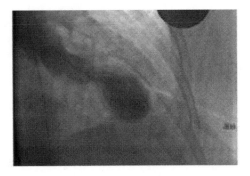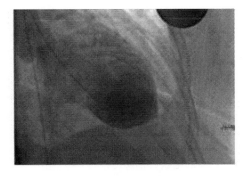

Figure 6.10: During systole, left ventricular angiography shows apical ballooning and hypercontraction of basal segments*. **Figure 6.11:** During diastole, it looks like normal*.

Diagnostic criteria: all of the following findings must be present for diagnoses:

- Transient hypokinesia, akinesia, or dyskinesia of the left ventricular mid segments with or without apical involvement. The regional wall motion abnormalities typically extend beyond a single epicardial coronary distribution. A stressful trigger is often, but not always, present.
- Absence of obstructive coronary disease or angiographic evidence of acute plaque rupture.
- New ECG abnormalities (either ST-segment elevation and/or T-wave inversion) or modest elevation in cardiac troponin.
- Absence of Pheochromocytoma or myocarditis.

MANAGEMENT

- Symptomatic
- Continue the standard regimen of MI until there is recovery of systolic function. Recovery takes 1-4 weeks in most cases.
- As this disease can recur, continue beta-blockers in the absence of contraindication.

HEART FAILURE

Heart failure is the inability of the heart to pump adequate amount of blood systematically to meet the demand of body.

It is broadly classified into 3 types:

- Left heart failure
- Right heart failure
- High output heart failure

LEFT HEART FAILURE

Left heart failure can be either due to systolic failure or diastolic failure.

SYSTOLIC HEART FAILURE

Systolic failure is due to the inability of the heart to contract efficiently. Heart is dilated and has high end systolic volume due to low ejection fraction.

Some major causes of systolic failure are: ischemic heart disease (most common), dilated cardiomyopathy, viral myocarditis, idiopathic myopathies in younger patients, peripartum cardiomyopathy.

DIASTOLIC HEART FAILURE

Diastolic failure is due to the inability of the heart to relax efficiently. Heart is stiffened and has normal or slightly high end systolic volume because contractility is not affected and ejection fraction is normal.

Some major causes of diastolic failure are: chronic hypertension (most common), hypertrophic cardiomyopathy, restrictive cardiomyopathies (amyloidosis, sarcoidosis, hemochromatosis).

CLINICAL PRESENTATION

- Patient often present with complaints of poor exercise tolerance resulting in shortness of breath, and easy fatigability.

- Paroxysmal nocturnal dyspnea: It is characterized by difficulty in breathing on laying down. Breathing difficulty occur due to the increase in venous return.

Standing up will decrease the venous return due to the pooling of blood in leg veins and therefore, the patient feels better in standing position.

- Physical exam findings may show inspiratory rales, peripheral ankle swelling, jugulovenous distension can be present if right-heart is involved.

- Fluid will leak out in the lung parenchyma due to increase in backward pressure in the pulmonary vessels. The characteristic of fluid is transudate. Peribronchiolar edema can narrow the airways, which will produce wheezes during expiration; this phenomenon is called as **cardiac asthma.**

- If pulmonary capillary ruptures, then heart failure cells can be found in the alveoli due to the hemosiderin endocytosis by alveolar macrophages.

- S3 heart sound can be heard in systolic failure due to rapid filling of ventricles in diastole. S4 heart sound can be heard in diastolic failure due to the atrial contraction against the stiffened ventricles.

New York Heart Association Classification

- Class I: No limitation of activities, no symptoms

- Class II: slight shortness of breath on moderate exertion, mild limitation of activities, comfortable with rest or with mild exertion

- Class III: marked limitation of activity, comfortable only at rest

  Class IV: confined to bed or chair, any physical activity brings discomfort. Uncomfortable even at rest.

DIAGNOSIS

- **BNP level:** the only use of BNP level is in an emergent situation when diagnosis of CHF is not clear.

  Normal BNP = No CHF. BNP test is highly sensitive but not specific.

  A high level cannot differentiate between systolic and diastolic failure.

If the BNP levels remain high after treatment – sign of bad prognosis.

- If BNP level is < 100 pg/mL = heart failure is highly unlikely.
- If BNP level is 100-500 pg/mL = results are uncertain but suspicious
- If BNP level is > 500 pg/ml = heart failure is highly likely.

False positive BNP test results for CHF include conditions that causes right or left ventricular stretching such as: pulmonary embolus, idiopathic pulmonary hypertension, cor pulmonale, renal failure, acute coronary syndrome, and cirrhosis. Rule out all possible causes of heart failure and perform essential diagnostic tests like ECG, Holter monitor, CBC, thyroid function test and other.

- **Chest x-ray:** will show cardiomegaly, Kerley B lines (septal edema), pulmonary vasculature congestion, air bronchogram.

- **ECG:** will show left ventricular hypertrophy (S wave in V1 + R in V5 or V6 > 35 mm)

- **Transthoracic echocardiography** (calculates the ejection fraction and valvular pathology).

- **Radionucleotide imaging** is most accurate but rarely used

MANAGEMENT

Treat the underlying cause of CHF if applicable. Salt restriction and lifestyle modification is recommended to everybody.

The primary goal for systolic failure is to decrease the afterload and preload. All of the following drugs are indicated in management of CHF unless contraindicated.

- **Diuretics**

  Loops diuretics like **furosemide** are preferred for systolic heart failure.

  They are not used if the patient is euvolemic in diastolic failure. It can be used in diastolic failure if the patient has volume overload/pulmonary edema but **avoid over-diuresis** because it will decrease the preload, thereby decreasing cardiac output and can lead to cardiogenic shock.

  Common findings of over-diuresis are dizziness, orthostatic hypotension, tachycardia, elevated creatinine, and activation of RAS system causing metabolic alkalosis.

- **ACE inhibitors or ARBs**

  ACE inhibitors are the most efficient group of drugs in systolic failure **with low ejection fraction**. It reduces both afterload and preload. If the patient develops cough and discomfort, switch ACE inhibitors to ARBs (receptor blocker)

- **Beta-blockers (metoprolol, carvedilol)**

  Beta-blockers are not the first line of drugs **in decompensated** systolic failure because beta-blockers are negative inotropic and further decreases stroke volume and worsens pulmonary edema.

  Beta-blocker can be considered in decompensated systolic failure after decreasing volume overload with diuretics (i.e. **for compensated** heart failure).

  Certain beta-blockers decrease mortality and therefore, given to everybody along with ACE inhibitors and diuretics unless contraindicated.

  They are the most efficient drugs in diastolic failure.

- **Aspirin:** it is indicated to every heart failure patient

- **Spironolactone or eplerenone**

  Spironolactone is used in NYHA class III and class IV heart failure after ACE inhibitors in patients with no hyperkalemia.

- **Combination of hydralazine and nitrates**

  Combination is used if the patient has hyperkalemia or rising creatinine level as a side effect of ACE inhibitors or ARBs. These combination is not beneficial in diastolic failure.

- **Inotropes (digoxin, milrinone, dobutamine)**

  Inotropes have no effect on mortality but they are used for symptomatic relief in NYHA class III and class IV systolic failure when ejection fraction is drastically low. They are not indicated in diastolic failure.

- **Implantable Cardioverter-Defibrillator (ICD) placement**

  ICD is indicated if the pharmacologic treatment fails and ejection fraction is less than 35% after 40 days of MI or 9 months for non-ischemic cardiomyopathy

- **Biventricular pacemaker defibrillator**

  If wide QRS (>120ms) and ejection fraction less than 35%. They improve both symptoms and mortality.

- **Heart transplantation** is the last choice if everything fails.

RIGHT HEART FAILURE

It is an inability of the right heart to pump out blood in the pulmonary circulation.

ETIOLOGY

- Left heart failure is the most common cause.

- Idiopathic pulmonary hypertension (BMPR2 mutation leading to pulmonary vasoconstriction).

- Pulmonary stenosis or embolization (give thrombolytic to break embolus in hemodynamically unstable patient).

- Right ventricular infarction (clear lungs, hypotension, JVD elevation).

- Restrictive cardiomyopathy, tricuspid, or pulmonary regurgitation.

- Congenital heart disease like atrial septal defect, ventricular septal defect, and tetralogy of fallot.

PHYSICAL FINDINGS

- Jugulovenous distension, peripheral edema (in ankle)
- Tricuspid valve regurgitation may be present or absent, S3-S4 sound on right side
- Fixed splitting (atrial septal defect)
- No crackles (if the right heart failure is not due to the left heart failure)
- Hepatosplenomegaly (zone 3 – central zone is affected most, ascites)
- Decrease in oxygen saturation will result in cyanosis

MANAGEMENT

- For isolated right heart failure due to right ventricular infarction, the best initial step in management is to give IV fluids to increase the preload because the right atrial pressure is high in right heart failure that decreases venous return to the heart. Giving IV fluids will increase pressure in the veins and venous return.

- Fluids are not indicated if right heart failure is associated with left heart failure or the patient has pulmonary crepitation (patient is already volume overloaded).

- If the patient does not respond, give dobutamine and then treat the underlying cause if possible. For RHF due to LHF, manage as like LHF, no fluids are given because they are already volume overloaded.

HIGH OUTPUT HEART FAILURE

High output failure is due to the persistent high cardiac output (high stroke volume)

ETIOLOGY

- Hyperthyroidism

- Severe anemia

- Thiamine deficiency (wet beriberi)

- Septic shock

- Arteriovenous fistula (trauma, shunt, Paget disease of bone)

- Obesity

CLINICAL PRESENTATION

- Breathlessness at rest or on exertion
- Exercise intolerance and fatigue
- The signs of typical heart failure may be present such as tachycardia, tachypnea, raised jugular pressure, pulmonary rales, pleural effusion, and peripheral edema.
- In high output heart failure, patients are likely to have warm rather than cold peripheries due to low systemic vascular resistance and peripheral vasodilatation.

PHYSICAL FINDINGS

- Examination of the systemic veins may reveal a cervical venous hum, heard best over the deep internal jugular veins, particularly on the right side. Less often, a venous hum may be appreciated over the femoral veins.

- Examination of the arteries may display signs related to increased left ventricular stroke volume. The pulse is usually bounding with a quick upstroke, and the pulse pressure is typically wide. Pistol-shot sounds may be auscultated over the femoral arteries, and a systolic bruit may be heard over the carotid arteries.

- Although these findings may be seen in other cardiac conditions, such as aortic regurgitation or patent ductus arteriosus, in the absence of these conditions, these signs are highly suggestive of elevated left ventricular stroke volume due to a hyperdynamic state.

DIAGNOSIS

- Echocardiography (best)
- Chest x-ray
- ECG
- Angiography to rule out any obstruction
- Thyroid function test

MANAGEMENT

- Clinical trial data in this area are lacking.

- The use of conventional therapies for heart failure, such as ACE inhibitors or ARBs, certain β-blockers and vasodilators are likely to further reduce systemic vascular resistance resulting in further deterioration.

- The condition, although uncommon, is often associated with a potentially correctable etiology. In the absence of a remediable cause, therapeutic options are very limited but include dietary restriction of salt and water combined with judicious use of diuretics.

- Vasodilators, β-agonist, inotropes are not recommended.

- IV vasoconstrictor adrenergic drugs like noradrenaline, ephedrine, and phenylephrine can be used for short time.

CARDIOMYOPATHY

Cardiomyopathy is the term applied to intrinsic disease of the cardiac muscle that produces myocardial dysfunction.

It is broadly classified into 3 types:

- Dilated cardiomyopathy
- Restrictive cardiomyopathy
- Hypertrophic cardiomyopathy

DILATED CARDIOMYOPATHY

Dilated cardiomyopathy results in systolic dysfunction. It is more common in young people.

ETIOLOGY

- Idiopathic
- Myocarditis
- Myocardial infarction
- Toxic exposures (alcohol)
- Wet beriberi (thiamine deficiency)
- Selenium deficiency
- Drugs like doxorubicin and daunorubicin
- Chagas disease (trypanosome cruzi)
- Pregnancy (peripartum)
- Myxedema (hypothyroidism)
- In 25%-35% cases genetic defects in cytoskeleton proteins

CLINICAL PRESENTATION

- Clinically presents with signs and symptoms of systolic heart failure.

- Shortness of breath, hypotension, rales, peripheral edema, raised JVP, and low ejection fraction can be present.

DIAGNOSIS

- Echocardiography is best, but order for ECG and chest x-ray also.

- ECG shows feature of atrial enlargement, low voltage QRS or left axis deviation.

- Interventricular conduction delays (bundle branch block) can occur due to cardiac dilation.

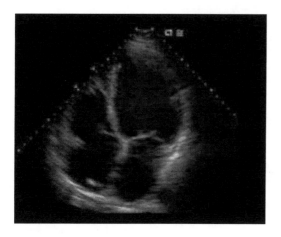

Figure 6.12: echocardiogram in dilated cardiomyopathy*.

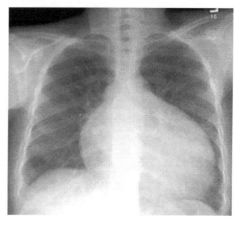

Figure 6.13: enlarged globular heart on chest x-ray*.

MANAGEMENT

- In addition to managing primary cause of dilated cardiomyopathy, diuretics with digoxin are frequently used to control the symptoms along with management of primary cause. Irreversible causes of dilated cardiomyopathy are managed same like systolic heart failure.

- If associated with left bundle branch block and patient is symptomatic, biventricular pacemaker or AICD (automated implantable cardioverter/defibrillator) is indicated.

RESTRICTIVE CARDIOMYOPATHY

Restrictive cardiomyopathy results in a stiff, noncompliant myocardium.

ETIOLOGY

- Infiltrative myopathy due to amyloidosis, sarcoidosis, hemochromatosis
- Enzyme deficiency – Pompe's disease (lysosomal alpha-glucosidase deficiency)
- Myocardial fibroelastosis

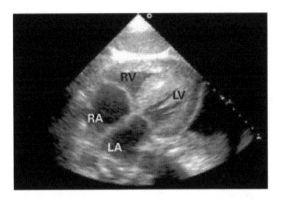

Figure 6.14: right and left ventricle walls are severely thickened*.

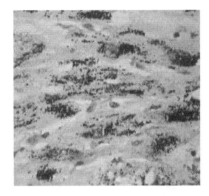

Figure 6.15: hemochromatosis

CLINICAL PRESENTATION

- Patient presents similarly like diastolic heart failure (discussed above).
- Shortness of breath, rales, peripheral edema, raised jugulovenous pressure, Normal ejection fraction.

DIAGNOSIS

- Echocardiography will clearly show thickened ventricles, but order for ECG and chest x-ray also. Biopsy is most definitive test.
- Rule out other possible causes like hemochromatosis, sarcoidosis, amyloidosis.

MANAGEMENT

- Manage the primary cause. If cause is unclear, it is managed like diastolic heart failure.

HYPERTROPHIC CARDIOMYOPATHY

Hypertrophic cardiomyopathy results in diastolic dysfunction of the heart.

The vast majority of cases are due to:

- Hypertension (most common): concentric hypertrophy in left ventricle, S4 gallop.

- Hypertrophic Obstructive Cardiomyopathy (HOCM): hypertrophy is more dominant at interventricular septum rather than left ventricle.

  This hypertrophy will obstruct the blood flow when preload decreases or peripheral vascular resistance is decreased (e.g. during exercise).

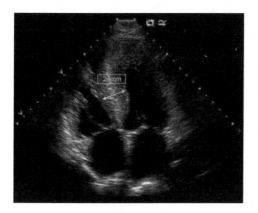

Figure 6.16: Interventricular septal hypertrophy

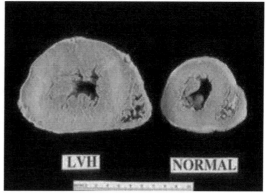

Figure 6.17: concentric hypertrophy*

HYPERTROPHIC OBSTRUCTIVE CARDIOMYOPATHY (HOCM)

- It is an autosomal dominant condition that occur due to the missense mutations in multiple genes encoding the contractile apparatus, in particular beta-myosin heavy chain.

- S4 gallop is not present. Signs of backward heart failure like pulmonary edema, right heart failure, and hepatomegaly is rarely present.

- HOCM is the main cause of sudden death in a healthy playing child.

CLINICAL PRESENTATION

- Dyspnea on heavy physical activity is the most common presentation

- Systolic crescendo-decrescendo murmur which is best heard at the left lower sternal border. Valsalva maneuver and changing position from squatting to standing will increase the intensity of the murmur.

- Angina or syncope with exercise

- Sudden death can occur due to ventricular arrhythmias

DIAGNOSIS

- Echocardiography is useful for diagnosis and many reveal normal ejection fraction and an asymmetrically thickening of ventricles.

  For a confirmatory diagnosis; a septum must be thickened 1.5 times of the posterior wall.

- If echocardiography is inconclusive, Cardiac Magnetic Resonance is indicated in patients with suspected HOCM.

- ECG, 24 hours Holter monitoring: to rule out ventricular tachycardia and determine whether the patient is a candidate for ICD therapy.

- Stress testing is done to determine functional capacity and response to therapy, for detection of exercise-induced left ventricular outflow obstruction.

MANAGEMENT

- No treatment is indicated if the patient is asymptomatic and septal thickness is lesser than 1.5 times posterior wall. Mild exercise is not contraindicated.

- If the interventricular septal thickness is greater 1.5 times, patient requires proper advice and treatment. Advise the patient to avoid heavy physical activity

- If the patients have dyspnea only, beta-blockers are the drug of choice. Beta-blockers will decrease the heart rate and increase preload by prolonging diastole.

  Verapamil can be used if beta-blocker therapy fails or contraindicated. Avoid verapamil in the setting of severe hypotension or dyspnea at rest.

- For management of acute hypotension, best initial step is to give IV fluids. If the fluids alone do not adequately control the blood pressure, IV phenylephrine is indicated.

- Diuretics are indicated for hypertrophy due to hypertension. No diuretics are indicated in the management of HOCM.

- Avoid inotropic drugs like digoxin, dobutamine, norepinephrine (increase in heart contractility might totally block outflow), vasodilators (reflex tachycardia) in HOCM.

- If the patient has an episode of syncope, implantable cardioversion or ablation/myomectomy is indicated.

Ablation of septum and Myomectomy in HOCM:

- In an ablation of septum, alcohol is injected in the hypertrophic muscle which leads to an infarction in that area, thereby reducing hypertrophy. It is only done when everything else fails or severe dyspnea or exertional syncope that interferes with daily life. It is considered a better choice in patients more than 40 years of age.

- Alcohol septal reduction is not done in patients younger than 21 years and is discouraged in adult less than 40 years if myomectomy is a possible option.

- Surgical myomectomy is the best treatment for HOCM however it is preferred at the first place in adults. It is considered a better choice in patients less than 40 years of age.

- It is more common among the people aged 15-40 years

PATHOGENESIS

- It is characterized by fibrofatty replacement of myocardial tissue in the right ventricle and fibrosis in the subepicardial region of the left ventricle. It is believed that the pathology has underlying desmosomal mutation.

CLINICAL PRESENTATION

- Often asymptomatic, with the first manifestation as sudden cardiac death.

- 2nd most common congenital cause of sudden death with exertions in young athletes (most common is HOCM).

- Palpitations, dyspnea, and syncope can be sometimes present.

DIAGNOSTIC CRITERIA

- Right ventricular dysfunction due to severe dilation and reduction of right ventricular ejection fraction with little or **no left ventricular impairment**, localized right ventricular aneurysms, severe segmental dilatation of the right ventricle.

- Regional right ventricular hypokinesia.

- **Tissue characterization:** fibrofatty replacement of myocardium on endomyocardial biopsy.
- **Conduction abnormalities:** epsilon waves in V_1 - V_3, localized prolongation (>110 ms) of QRS in V_1 - V_3, frequent premature ventricular contractions.
- Family history of sudden death < 35 years that was confirmed on autopsy or surgery.

DIAGNOSIS

- ECG (nonspecific T-wave inversion in V1-V3), epsilon wave (small upstroke after QRS complex) can be seen in 50% of ARVC).

- Echocardiography will show enlarged, hypokinetic, thin right ventricle, cardiac MRI, biopsy.

- Right ventricular angiography and biopsy.

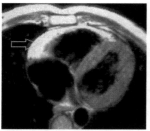

Figure 6.18: RV wall with the fatty replacement of myocardium.

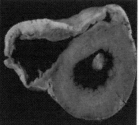

Figure 6.19: RV dilation with anterior & posterior aneurysms*

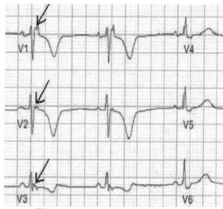

Figure 6.20: epsilon wave

MANAGEMENT

- Management depends on the diagnostic findings and clinical presentation. The aim is to decrease sudden cardiac death,

- Heart transplantation is the best treatment.

- Anti-arrhythmic (sotalol – class 3 anti-arrhythmic), anticoagulants, catheter ablation or implantation of defibrillators can help temporarily. The disease is genetic and progressive.

THUNDERNOTE: NAXOS DISEASE and CARVAJAL SYNDROME

(very unlikely to be tested on USMLE)

- An autosomal recessive variant of ARVC with wooly hair and palmoplantar keratoma.

- It can be seen in Immigrant from Turkey, Israel, Saudi Arabia, India and Ecuador

- The pathogenesis behind naxos disease is the deletion in plakoglobin gene [cell adhesion protein].

- **Carvajal syndrome** is a variant of Naxos disease that more **commonly involves left heart.** They have mutation in desmoplakin gene [also a cell adhesion gene] and it manifest as dilated cardiomyopathy in early childhood)

CLINICAL PRESENTATION

- Wooly hair at birth

- Palmoplantar keratoma can appear during the first year of life

- Signs of **right heart failure** in late stages during childhood (ARVC)

DIAGNOSIS

- ECG, Echocardiography (similar to ARVC)

- **Biopsy:**
  In Naxos disease; loss of **right** ventricular myocardium with fibrofatty replacement.
  In Carvajal disease; loss of **left** ventricular myocardium with fibrosis (no fatty component).

MANAGEMENT

- Implantation of automatic cardioverter defibrillator is indicated to prevent sudden death.

- Pharmacological and antiarrhythmic management of congestive heart failure and ventricular tachycardia.

- Heart transplantation is best.

PERIPARTUM CARDIOMYOPATHY

- A form of dilated cardiomyopathy.

- It is the worst cardiac disease in a pregnant woman. Eisenmenger syndrome is the second worst.

- Cardiac function begins deteriorating typically between the last month of pregnancy to 6-months postpartum.

- Peripartum cardiomyopathy is a diagnosis of exclusion, wherein patients have no prior history of heart disease and there are no other known possible causes of heart failure.

ETIOLOGY

- Causes of peripartum cardiomyopathy are unknown.

- It is believed to occur due to enormous production of antibodies against myocardium.

- Possible causes of these antibodies include cardiotropic viruses, selenium deficiency, and genetics.

- Advice the woman to not become pregnant, because If she does, there will be severe flare of postpartum cardiomyopathy which can be fatal.

PATHOGENESIS

- An inflammatory process is initiated in the heart due to the enormous production of antibodies. Consequently, heart muscle cells are damaged; some die or become scar tissue.

- Scar tissue has no ability to contract; therefore, the effectiveness of the pumping action of the heart is decreased. In addition, damage to the cytoskeletal framework of the heart will lead to enlargement of the heart that decreases its systolic function resulting in low cardiac output.

- Progressive loss of heart muscle cells will eventually lead to heart failure. Most left ventricular dysfunction does not rich till this stage and is short-term and reversible.

- There is an increase in the risk of atrioventricular arrhythmias, thromboembolism and even sudden cardiac death.

DIAGNOSIS

- An echocardiogram is used to both diagnose and monitor the effectiveness of treatment for PPCM.

Focused medical history for PPCM screening looking for early symptoms of heart failure during last month of pregnancy		
	1 Point	2 Point
Orthopnea	Need to elevate head	Need to elevate upper body 45' or more
Dyspnea	Climbing 8 or more steps	Walking on level
Unexplained Cough	Night time	Day and night
Peripheral pitting edema	Below knee	Above and below knee and/or hands/face
Weight gain during last month of pregnancy	2-4 lbs per week	Over 4 lbs per week
Palpitation	When lying down at night	Day and night, any position

Scoring and risk evaluation:

- 0 - 2 = low risk: continue observation

- 3 - 4 = mild risk: consider doing blood BNP and CRP. Echocardiography is indicated if BNP and CRP are elevated.

- 5 or more = high risk: do blood BNP, CRP, and echocardiogram

Table 6.3: risk evaluation for peripartum cardiomyopathy

MANAGEMENT

- Manage it like a congestive heart failure with ACE inhibitors or ARBs, beta-blockers, spironolactone, diuretics, digoxin. **ACE inhibitors** are indicated **after the delivery.**

- If ejection fraction is less than 40%, anticoagulation is required because there is a greater risk of developing left ventricular thrombi.

- Sometimes implantation of a Left Ventricular Assist Device (LVAD) or even heart transplant may also become necessary.

- The survival rate is 98% or better. Almost all patients improve with treatment.

- Patient is advised to avoid another pregnancy if ejection fraction is less than 55%. Once fully recovered, if there is no subsequent pregnancy, the possibility of relapse or recurrence of heart failure is minimal.

THUNDERNOTE: CAUSES OF PERIPHERAL EDEMA	
Increase in capillary hydrostatic pressure	Due to an increase in flow as a result of vasodilation Due to an increase in capillary pressure (venous obstruction, CHF) Due to an increase in blood volume (hypotonic infusions)
Decrease in vascular pressure	Due to damage in the liver and kidney (nephrotic syndrome, liver cirrhosis)
Increase in capillary permeability	Due to an inflammation (TNF-alpha, histamine, bradykinin) Due to cancer therapy (interleukin-2 is associated with pulmonary edema)
Lymphedema	Due to filariasis (Wucheria bancrofti causes elephantiasis), bacterial lymphangitis (streptococcus), trauma, surgery (radical mastectomy), tumor

Table 6.4: causes of edema

CIRCULATORY SHOCK

Circulatory shock is a medical emergency that occurs due to an inadequacy of oxygen for oxidative phosphorylation.

CLINICAL PRESENTATION

- Sudden fall in blood pressure (chronic hypertensive can have higher pressure than normotensive).
- Reduced mean arterial pressure < 60 mmHg.
- Tachycardia, tachypnoea.
- Cool skin and extremities and low urine output.
- Confusion or loss of consciousness (due to under perfusion of end organs).
- Lactic acidosis will occur due to tissue hypoxia.
- Very high mortality rate, if not treated immediately.

End organ damage can occur such as:

- Kidney: acute tubular necrosis, electrolyte abnormalities
- Brain: ischemic encephalopathy
- Heart: widespread coagulative necrosis, contraction band necrosis
- Gastrointestinal: patchy necrosis and hemorrhage (hemorrhagic enteropathy), fatty liver

Incidence rate in ICU:

- Septic shock (more than 55% cases, causes vasodilation and will have warm extremities)
- Cardiogenic shock and hypovolemic shock (around 15-20%)
- Obstructive shock is very rare

PATHOGENESIS

- **Early stage (non-progressive):** compensatory mechanisms will help to increase end organ perfusion by increasing RAAS system and SNS activity (increases heart rate, peripheral vasoconstriction, and renal fluid conservation).

- **Progressive stage:** compensatory mechanisms are not adequate which will result in tissue hypoperfusion resulting in renal insufficiency, circulatory and metabolic imbalances such as lactic acidosis. Once progressive stage starts, it rapidly moves to an irreversible stage.

- **Irreversible stage:** end organ damage and metabolic disturbances that are incompatible with life such as renal shutdown, myocardial infarction, and neuronal damage.

CLASSIFICATION

Cardiogenic shock:

- Due to primary pathology in the heart that decreases cardiac output – cardiac tamponade and tension pneumothorax.

- Other conditions that can cause shock like situation are left ventricular dysfunction (arrhythmias, MI, valvular heart disease, myocarditis).

- Blood pools up backward leading to pulmonary congestion.

Obstructive shock:

- Sudden decrease in cardiac output due to pulmonary embolus, cardiac tamponade, or tension pneumothorax.

- When presented acutely, you should not wait for any investigation like chest x-ray, ECG or anything else.

- Next best step in acute setting is needle decompression for tamponade or tension pneumothorax, or position change for air embolus.

Hypovolemic shock:

- Due to acute loss of blood volume (severe internal or external hemorrhage from trauma or excessive burn, severe vomiting and diarrhea).

- Hypovolemic shock is differentiated from cardiogenic shock by the single most finding of low central venous pressure resulting in collapsed/empty neck vein. The cardiogenic shock will have high central venous pressure due to backward congestion of blood resulting in distended neck vein.

- If the source of bleeding is external, first stop the bleeding by compression and then ask your fellow to perform ABC.

Distributive shock:

- Due to release of inflammatory mediators - includes septic and anaphylactic shock

- **Septic shock** is the most common cause of death in ICU. It is a systemic response to severe infection most commonly due to gram-negative bacteria (endotoxin-mediated or superantigen-mediated toxic shock syndrome). Endotoxin activates WBC and endothelium. Mild amount of endotoxin will cause fever and other systemic effect. The high amount of endotoxin will lead to the release of acute phase reactants like IL 1, IL 6, IL 8, TNF-Alpha.

- The acute phase reactants will cause severe vasodilation leading to peripheral pooling of blood, endothelial injury leading to Disseminated Intravascular Coagulation (DIC) or Acute Respiratory Distress Syndrome (ARDS) due to alveolar capillary damage)

- **Anaphylactic shock** occurs due to sudden and severe vasodilation due to allergic reaction or transfusion reaction such as ABO-incompatibility. Immediate epinephrine is the best therapy followed by ABC regimen.

Neurogenic shock:

- Occurs usually due to the trauma that interrupts sympathetic vasomotor outflow that leads to severe vasodilation.

DIAGNOSIS

- History and physical findings

- In suspected cardiogenic shock, focused echocardiography is performed as soon as possible to assess various factors like left ventricular size, pericardial effusions, and stroke volume.

- High level of lactate is generally present due to anaerobic metabolism by the tissue.

MANAGEMENT

- Start resuscitation even before various investigations.
- Once identified, the cause must be corrected rapidly (e.g. control of bleeding, percutaneous coronary intervention for coronary syndromes, thrombolysis or embolectomy for massive pulmonary embolism, and administration of antibiotics and source control for septic shock).

Initial resuscitation in circulatory shock:

Check whether airways are clear and then VIP

- Ventilate (oxygen administration)
- Infuse (fluid resuscitation), and
- Pump (administration of vasoactive agents)
- Insert arterial catheter for monitoring of arterial blood pressure and blood sampling, plus a central venous catheter for the infusion of fluids and vasoactive agents and to guide fluid therapy.

Indications for endotracheal intubation:

- Severe dyspnea

- Hypoxemia

- Persistent or worsening acidemia (pH <7.30)

Fluids for resuscitation:

- Crystalloid: normal saline is generally preferred as the first choice in fluid administration (300-500 ml fluid in 20 minutes or 1-2L as fast as it can go). Reassess the patient to determine whether bolus has helped or not. A positive sign is an increase in blood pressure and urine output. Give the second bolus if the first bolus leads no improvement. Pulmonary edema and CHF are the most serious complication. Foley catheter should be placed to ensure accurate monitoring of urine output.

- Colloids are 2nd choice due to high cost. Both crystalloids and colloids are equally efficacious.

Drugs for resuscitation:

- In the absence of left ventricular outflow tract obstruction, **norepinephrine or dobutamine** is indicated if the fluids alone fail to control hypotension.

- Pure alpha agonist like phenylephrine or nonselective beta-agonist like isoproterenol is not indicated due to a potential side effect.

- Norepinephrine will increase the cardiac output by its action on beta-1 receptor. In addition, it will also cause peripheral vasoconstriction by its alpha-1 action, which will deviate the circulatory blood to the vital organs.

- Epinephrine is 2nd line drug in circulatory shock management due to a potential risk of beta-2 receptor-mediated vasodilator activity (1st for an anaphylactic shock because the beta-2 action of epinephrine will also cause bronchial dilation).

- Dobutamine or other ionotropic agents are not indicated if the hypotension/shock is due to the left ventricular outflow tract obstruction because they will worsen the situation.

- Recommended approach for the patient with moderate-to-severe LVOT obstruction includes the use of beta blockers.

ACUTE CARDIAC TAMPONADE

- Cardiac tamponade is mainly differentiated from tension pneumothorax based on breath sounds.

- In tamponade bilateral breath sound will be present while in tension pneumothorax they will be absent on affected side (trachea deviates to the opposite side).

- Beck's triad is classic for tamponade: hypotension + distended neck vein + muffled heart sound.

- Acute management is needle through the xiphoid process into the cardiac space and aspirate the blood. Then go to the surgery and close the hole that had resulted in tamponade.

- Chest compressions are indicated if the patient is not stable and have systolic pressure < 70 mmHg.

TENSION PNEUMOTHORAX

- In tension pneumothorax, the best next step is needle decompression at 2nd intercostal space at midclavicular line and then place a chest tube.

- Decompression is done on the opposite side of trachea deviation, for e.g. if trachea had deviated to the right, absent breath sound will be on the left side and decompression is done on the left side.

- Tracheal intubation is contraindicated in tension pneumothorax or in flail chest (multiple adjacent rib fractures).

- Do prophylactic insertion of chest tube on both sides in any patient with flail chest.

- Chest tube placement is done at 5th intercostal space at anterior axillary even for hemothorax and pyothorax.

PULMONARY AIR EMBOLISM

- Any penetrating injury to neck or chest can cause an air embolism. This embolus will travel through the veins to the right ventricle and if the embolus is large enough to obstruct the outflow of right ventricles, sudden death can occur.

- Physical findings are distended neck veins and sloshing heart sounds (sound like air and water are mixing – blow air through pipe into the water and the sound that comes when bubble burst is a sloshing sound)

- Immediately turn the patients head down with the right side up, do not wait even for a blink of an eye. This position of the patient will help the air bubble to rise up (toward the apex of heart) and thus opens up the right ventricular obstruction. Then close the source of air embolus.

MYOCARDITIS

Myocarditis is an inflammation in myocardium without the blockage of coronary arteries or other common noninfectious causes.

ETIOLOGY

- Infections like adenovirus, Group B coxsackievirus, parvovirus (lymphocytic infiltrate), Lyme disease, diphtheria toxin, Trichinella spiralis and others.

  Streptococcal M protein, diphtheria toxin, and Coxsackie B virus have epitopes that are immunologically similar to cardiac myosin. This leads to cross-reaction between the immune system and myocardium.

- Bites: black widow spider bite and scorpion bite.

- Drugs: doxorubicin, zidovudine (oxidative damage).

- Autoimmune disease: SLE is the most common cause in an autoimmune disease, Kawasaki disease.

CLINICAL PRESENTATION

- Symptomatic cases can present with shortness of breath, fever, mild stabbing chest pain (if associated with concurrent pericarditis), palpitations, or syncope.

- Sudden cardiac death can occur due to underlying ventricular arrhythmias or atrioventricular block.

- **Sarcoid myocarditis:** lymphadenopathy, arrhythmias, sarcoid involvement in other organs (up to 70%), hypercalcemia, elevate ACE level (the cells surrounding granulomas can produce increased amounts of **ACE** and the blood **level** of **ACE** may increase when **sarcoidosis** is present).

- **Acute rheumatic fever:** usually affects the heart in 50-90%; associated signs, such as erythema marginatum, polyarthralgia, chorea, subcutaneous nodules (Jones criteria) can be present.

- **Hypersensitive/eosinophilic myocarditis:** pruritic maculopapular rash and history of using offending drug.

- **Giant cell myocarditis:** sustained ventricular tachycardia in rapidly progressive heart failure. AV block can also occur with giant cell myocarditis.

- **Peripartum cardiomyopathy:** heart failure developing in the last month of pregnancy or within 6 months following delivery.

DIAGNOSIS

- Myocarditis will always have an underlying primary cause and diagnose is usually presumptive based on history. Rule out other serious conditions.
- Chest x-ray, echocardiogram
- ECG may show diffuse T wave inversions, saddle-shaped ST-segment elevations. Such findings are also present in pericarditis.
- MRI can help to confirm diagnose of myocarditis.
- CBC (elevated CRP, ESR). Increase in cardiac enzymes like troponin and CK-MB (a normal value does not exclude myocarditis).
- Cardiac catheterization and endomyocardial biopsy – gold standard test, but invasive approach limits its usage.

MANAGEMENT

- Treat the underlying cause

- Rest and reducing the workload on your heart is an important part of recovery.

- Myocarditis can give rise to acute heart failure or evolve into dilated cardiomyopathy. If myocarditis is associated with heart failure, treat like CHF (ACEi/ARB, diuretics, beta-blockers)

If the patient's condition does not improve after primary managements and patient is unstable, temporary artificial heart (ventricular assist device) and intra-aortic balloon pump can be considered.

- Intra-aortic balloon pump: a balloon is surgically inserted into the aorta. As the balloon inflates and deflates, it will help to increase cardiac output and decrease the workload on the heart.

- Extracorporeal membrane oxygenation: This device helps to Increase the oxygen content of the blood. When blood is removed from the body, it passes through a special membrane in the ECMO machine that removes carbon dioxide and adds oxygen to the blood. The newly oxygenated blood is then returned to the body. The ECMO machine takes over the work of the heart. This treatment is used to allow the heart to recover or while waiting for other treatments, such as heart transplant.

- If everything fails and still arrhythmia persists: heart transplantation is required.

CARDIAC CONTUSION

Cardiac contusion is defined as a bruise in the myocardium. It is most commonly associated with the trauma of anterior chest wall like flail chest.

A right heart is more commonly affected because of its anatomic location as the most anterior surface of heart.

Clinical presentation: pain in front of the ribs or sternum, palpitations, light-headedness, nausea and vomiting, shortness of breath and fatigue. When myocardial contusion is suspected, look for the aortic dissection.

Complication: arrhythmia (most common), myocardial infarction, rupture or cardiogenic shock.

Management: Screening strategy to identify patient at risk for cardiac complication in relation to the severity of associated injuries:

- If the patient is hemodynamically unstable with multiple trauma, admit to ICU and perform transthoracic echo or transesophageal echo.

- If the patient is hemodynamically stable with suspected sternal fracture and associated injury, admit to ICU and perform transthoracic echo or transesophageal echo to rule out aortic injuries.

- If the patient is hemodynamically stable with elevated cardiac enzymes and ECG abnormalities but no signs of sternal fracture, admit the patient in hospital for cardiac observation and monitoring. Serial ECGs and troponin levels are measured. If the clinical status of patient deteriorates, perform transthoracic or transesophageal echocardiography.

- If the patient has mild injury with normal ECG and cardiac enzymes, perform follow up ECG within 24 hours. No hospital admission is required in mild injury. If significant changes are present on ECG during follow up, admit the patient to the hospital for cardiac observation and monitoring. If the clinical status deteriorates, perform transthoracic or transesophageal echocardiography.

- Pericarditis is an inflammation of the pericardium.
- Dense scar tissue with dystrophic calcification can lead to constrictive pericarditis where the heart chambers fail to dilate.

CLINICAL PRESENTATION

- Fever, tachycardia

- Chest pain is relieved by leaning forward. Pain does not change with respirations. Pain with pleural friction rub increases with inspiration.

- Pericardial friction rub is heard during systole, early and late diastole.

- Cardiac enzymes are increased in 40% cases where pericarditis is associated with myocarditis.

ETIOLOGY

- **Acute pericarditis** tends to occur around 2-3 days following a transmural MI is common.

- **Dressler's syndrome** tends to occur around 2-6 weeks following an MI. The underlying pathophysiology is thought to be an autoimmune reaction against antigenic proteins formed as the myocardium recovers.

- **Viral pericarditis:** Coxsackievirus and echovirus are the most common cause of acute pericarditis. Viral pericarditis is more common in the young person with a history of a recent upper respiratory infection, low-grade fever, pleuritic chest pain that changes with position, and a pericardial friction rub (the scratchy sound).

- In acute bacterial pericarditis, the exudate is fibrinopurulent.

- **Pericarditis with malignancy** is associated with fibrinous exudate and bloody effusion.

- **Tuberculous pericarditis** shows the area of caseation. When there is excessive suppuration or caseation then healing occurs by fibrosis (chronic pericarditis). This fibrotic tissue obliterates pericardial space.

- **Uremic pericarditis:** Patient with the chronic renal disease can develop uremic pericarditis, after missing multiple dialysis session. It can ultimately result in pericardial fluid accumulation and cardiac tamponade.

DIAGNOSIS

- Patient presenting with classic presentation of pericarditis must be given NSAIDs unless contraindicated before establishing the diagnosis. NSAIDs are not indicated in acute pericarditis after an MI.

- Chest x-ray is the best initial test in patient presenting with pleuritic chest pain. water bottle configuration indicates the presence of effusion.

- ECG will show diffuse ST elevation in all leads with PR depression (classic for pericarditis).

- Echocardiography

- Cardiac MRI

MANAGEMENT

- Treat the primary cause.

- For viral or idiopathic pericarditis give NSAIDS like Ibuprofen, Naproxen, Indomethacin.

- Avoid NSAIDs in post-MI pericarditis because it will interfere with the scar formation.

- Colchicine decreases recurrence.

- Use steroids if NSAIDs fails.

- In TB pericarditis or constrictive pericarditis, pericardial resection might be required.

- Pericardiocentesis if an effusion is present.

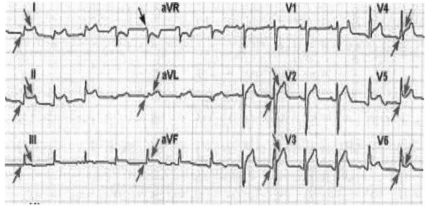

Figure 6.21: Diffuse ST elevation with PR depression*

In extreme cases, the heart is completely encased by dense fibrosis that it cannot expand normally during diastole so-called constrictive pericarditis. It can be due to any cause of pericarditis (discussed in previous topic). Tuberculosis is the most common cause.

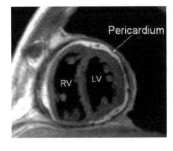
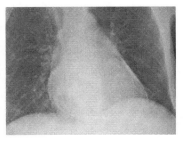
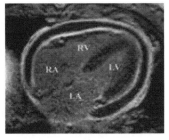

Figure 6.22: layer of calcification surrounding the heart*

Figure 6.23: white calcific line surrounding the heart*

Figure 6.24: High intense 2 layers indicate inflammation + black area between the 2 layers indicates pericardial effusion (fibrinous pericarditis)*

CLINICAL PRESENTATION

- Patient with constrictive pericarditis typically presents with features of right heart failure such as shortness of breath and elevated JVP

- Ascites and edema due to hepatomegaly

- Pericardial knock and loud S3 can be heard on auscultation

- Kussmaul's sign: It is a reflection of blood into the jugular vein on inspiration. Compression created by calcified pericardium decreases venous return to the heart during inspiration.

DIAGNOSIS

- Chest x-ray is the best initial test. A layer of calcification is seen surrounding the heart.

- Echocardiography

- CT or MRI

MANAGEMENT

- Pericardial resection is the best treatment.

CARDIAC TAMPONADE

Cardiac tamponade occurs due to the accumulation of fluid or blood in the pericardial cavity. The rate of fluid accumulation is the most important prognostic factor in determining the severity of cardiac tamponade.

ETIOLOGY

- Dissecting aortic aneurysm (thoracic)
- End-stage lung cancer
- Acute MI
- Heart surgery
- Bacterial or viral pericarditis

CLINICAL PRESENTATION

Rapid accumulation of fluid in the pericardial cavity can presents with features of shock. Immediate pericardiocentesis required if the patient is hemodynamically unstable and cardiac tamponade is suspected.

Slow accumulation of fluid in the pericardium over the period of time does not present with sudden hemodynamic instability because it gives enough time to the heart to get stretched. They more often present with features of pericardial effusion such as:

- Shortness of breath and clear lungs.

- Muffled heart sound - difficult to hear due to the fluid surrounding the heart.

- Hypotension: Equalization of pressure in all chambers and failure in relaxation of right heart decreases preload and cardiac output.

- **Pulsus paradoxus** is a drop in systolic blood pressure by >10 mmHg during inspiration. Dilation of pulmonary arteries during inspiration lead to an increase in venous return to the right heart. The high pressure generated by increase in venous return to the right ventricle pushes the interventricular septum to the left and decreases left ventricular cavity size during diastole. This results in low preload, low stroke volume and fall in blood pressure by > 10mmHg.

DIAGNOSIS

- Chest x-ray shows globular heart (enlarged heart in both left and right direction).

- ECG - low voltage and electrical alternans (different heights of QRS complex),

- Echocardiography is needed to confirm diagnoses. It will show fluid in the pericardial cavity and failure in right heart relaxation.

- Angiography, CT or MRI of the chest. Tamponade and constrictive pericarditis are not differentiated by catheterization.

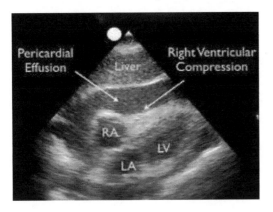

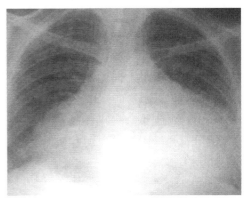

Figure 6.25: Pericardial effusion compressing right ventricular during diastole*

Figure 6.26: massive cardiomegaly and normal lung field due to massive pericardial effusion*

MANAGEMENT

- Cardiac tamponade is an emergency condition that needs to be treated in the hospital. The first step of management is to drain the fluid from the pericardial cavity of the heart.

- If the patient is hemodynamically unstable, acute management is needle through the xiphoid process into the cardiac space and aspirate the blood. Then go to the surgery and close the hole that had resulted in tamponade. Pericardiectomy may also be done.

- For recurrent cases, place a hole or window into the pericardium.

- Diuretics are not prescribed. Fluids are given to keep blood pressure normal until the fluid can be drained surrounding the heart. Drugs that increase blood pressure may also help keep the person alive until the fluid is drained.

- Chest compressions are indicated if the patient is not stable and have systolic pressure < 70 mmHg. Oxygen may be given to help reduce the workload on the heart by decreasing tissue demands for blood flow. The primary cause of tamponade must be identified and treated.

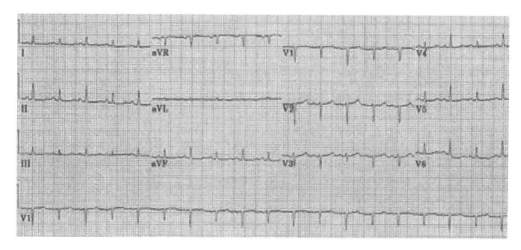

Figure 6.27: QRS alternans (different amplitude of QRS complexes)

	Cardiac tamponade	Constrictive pericarditis
JVP (normal)	Absent Y-descent	Steep Y-descent
Pulsus paradoxus	Present	Absent
Kussmaul's sign	Rare	Present
Pericardial calcification	Absent (if primary cause is not a constrictive pericarditis)	Present

Table 6.5: differences between constrictive pericarditis and cardiac tamponade

Evaluation of the patient with suspected valvular heart disease:

- Careful history and physical examination
- ECG is done to check for heart rhythm.
- Chest x-ray is done to assess the presence or absence of pulmonary congestion and other lung pathology.
- Transthoracic echocardiogram (TTE) is the best initial test when valvular lesions are suspected. It is done to assess the effect of the valvular lesion on cardiac chambers and other concomitant valve lesions.

Other ancillary testing that can be ordered in selective patients are:

- Transesophageal echocardiography (TEE) is even more sensitive and specific than transthoracic echocardiography but the sensitivity of TTE is 95% which is high enough to rule out valvular disease. If TTE is inconclusive and valvular disease is suspected, then TEE is indicated.
- CT or Cardiac Magnetic Resonance, stress testing and cardiac catheterization (most accurate) may be required to determine optimal treatment.
- Cardiac catheterization is recommended in symptomatic patients when non-invasive tests are inconclusive or when there is a discrepancy between the severity of disease on non-invasive testing and physical examination.
- Exercise testing is reasonable in selected patients with asymptomatic severe valvular disease to assess the hemodynamic response to exercise and to determine next step in management.
- All patients who had been diagnosed with the valvular disease should also undergo guideline-determined therapy for other comorbidities like hypertension, diabetes, and hypercholesterolemia.

Periodic monitoring with transthoracic echo is recommended in asymptomatic patients with known valvular heart disease depending on valve lesion, severity, ventricular size, and function.

- **Mild:** every 3-5 years
- **Moderate (progressive):** every 1-2 years
- **Severe:** every 6-12 months

THUNDERNOTE: Cardiac Catheterization

- Cardiac catheterization is performed to further evaluate coronary artery disease, valvular heart disease, congestive heart failure, and/or certain congenital heart conditions when other less invasive diagnostic tests indicate the presence of one of these conditions. It is **never** the first choice for any condition

- In cardiac catheterization, a very small hollow tube, or catheter, is advanced from a blood vessel in the groin or arm through the aorta into the heart. Once the catheter is in place, several diagnostic techniques may be used.

- The tip of the catheter can be placed into various parts of the heart to measure the pressures within the chambers.

- **Coronary angiography:** the catheter can be advanced into the coronary arteries and a contrast dye is injected into the arteries. It aims to detect any narrowing of the coronary arteries, the exact site and severity of any narrowing.

- Angioplasty, Percutaneous Coronary Intervention, and stenting may be done as part of, or following a catheterization.

- Biopsy: a small sample of heart tissue may be obtained during the procedure to be examined later under the microscope for abnormalities.

The person will remain awake during the procedure although a small amount of sedating medication will be given prior to the procedure to ensure the patient remains comfortable during the procedure.

Complication: Cardiac tamponade, injury to a coronary artery and MI, arrhythmia, hypotension, stroke (post-embolectomy), and renal insufficiency due to the contrast dye (more common in patients with diabetes or kidney problems)

Contraindication: Renal Insufficiency, high fever, coagulopathy, cardiac myxoma, uncontrolled arrhythmias, hypertensive crisis, and uncompensated heart failure

INFECTIVE ENDOCARDITIS

- Infective endocarditis is due to infection of the endocardial surface of the heart, which may include one or more heart valves, the mural endocardium, or a septal defect.

- Intra-cardiac effects of endocarditis include severe valvular insufficiency that may lead to intractable congestive heart failure and myocardial abscesses.

- If left untreated, infective endocarditis is generally fatal.

- Most common and strongest risk factor for endocarditis is previously damaged valves.

ETIOLOGY

- Rheumatic heart disease (mitral valve, aortic valve)

- Congenital heart disease (ASD, VSD, TOF)

- Prosthetic valve (S. aureus is most common, S. epidermitis, candida)

- IV Drug user (S. aureus is most common, Pseudomonas, right sided lesions)

- S. viridans (on previously injured endocardium, most common cause of **subacute endocarditis**, 40-50% cases). S. aureus and group B strep have the highest mortality rates.

- Enterococci (most common in indwelling urinary catheters)

- Streptococcus bovis (check for colon cancer).

- Bartonella quintana must be considered in cases of culture-negative endocarditis among homeless individuals, Transmitted by flea bite.

- Coxiella Q is more common in culture-negative endocarditis than HACEK organisms. HACEK: Hemophilus, Actinobacillus, Cardiobacterium, Eikenella, Kingella

- Fungal endocarditis (candida and aspergillus)

- Nosocomial (IV catheters, pacemakers, and defibrillators, hemodialysis shunts, chemotherapeutic and hyperalimentation lines – most common cause of increased incidence over the past years.

- Non-bacterial thrombotic endocarditis - SLE (Libman-Sacks endocarditis, sterile vegetations over mitral valve)

- Malignancy - marantic endocarditis (sterile, possible pathogenesis is procoagulant effect of circulating mucin from mucin-producing tumors of colon or pancreas. Non-destructive vegetations are formed on cardiac valves and act as a nidus for infections).

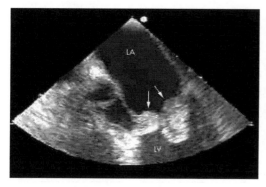 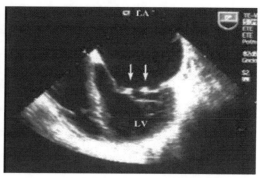

Figure 6.28: large vegetations of IE*   **Figure 6.29:** small vegetations of NBTE (Libman-sacks endocarditis)*

VALVE INVOLVEMENT

- The majority of infective endocarditis involves left valves (90% cases).
- The mitral valve is most commonly involved on the left side.
- IV drug users will have involvement of right-sided valves (tricuspid valve most common).
- Vegetation of infective endocarditis is large and can damage the valvular structure.
- Vegetation of non-bacterial thrombotic endocarditis are small and sterile (due to hypercoagulable state and not due to inflammation), damages valve over a long period of time.

PATHOGENESIS

- Previously damaged valves will have reactive endothelial cells that are vulnerable to inflammatory mediators. This lead to platelet and fibrin adherence at the damaged area.
- Sometimes bacteria get entrapped in this process and hide from body's immune system. They proliferate inside the entrapped area, lay down more fibrin and form vegetation.
- This vegetation destroys the valve leaflet or chordae tendinae, which will lead to regurgitant murmurs.

CLINICAL PRESENTATION

- low-grade fever is present in 90% cases of IE.

- New onset murmur with changing intensity in acute IE.

  Right-sided murmur increases with inspiration. Left sided murmur decreases with inspiration. The right-sided lesion can give an embolic phenomenon in the lungs. Multiple micro-abscesses in lungs indicates right sided endocarditis.

- Osler nodes: painful nodules on pads of finger or toes due to embolization of bacteria encoded in vegetation. Over the period of time, these nodules become sterile and develop vasculitis in surrounding areas.

- Janeway lesion: painless area of hemorrhage on palms and soles.

- Splinter hemorrhages: linear hemorrhage in nail beds

- Roth's spots: retinal hemorrhage with small, clear center (very rare)

- Systemic embolization: clinical presentation depends upon the location of emboli; for e.g. focal neurologic deficits or acute mesenteric ischemia.

- Subacute bacterial endocarditis: symptoms are mild and nonspecific; weeks to months of low-grade fever, malaise, weight loss, flu-like symptoms, symptoms of systemic emboli.

- Non-bacterial endocarditis: usually asymptomatic but it can cause heart failure by destroying valves. Other findings such as glomerulonephritis, arthritis and skin rash can be present if it is associated with SLE or other immune-complex disease.

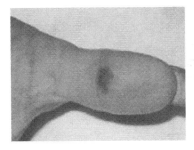

Figure 6.30: Osler node*

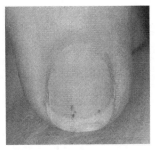

Figure 6.31: splinter hemorrhage*

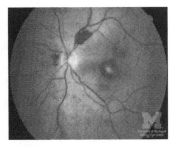

Figure 6.32: Roth spots

DUKE'S DIAGNOSTIC CRITERIA

Major criteria:

- Two blood cultures positive for organisms typically found in patients with IE. Three or more separate blood cultures were drawn at least 1 hour apart.

- Echocardiogram positive for IE, documented by an oscillating intra-cardiac mass on a valve or on supporting structures.

- Myocardial abscess

- Development of partial dehiscence of a prosthetic valve

- New-onset valvular regurgitation

Minor criteria:

- Predisposing heart condition or intravenous drug use

- Fever of 38°C (100.4°F) or higher

- Vascular phenomenon, including major arterial emboli, septic pulmonary infarcts, mycotic aneurysm, intracranial hemorrhage, conjunctival hemorrhage, or Janeway lesions

- Immunologic phenomena such as glomerulonephritis, Osler nodes, Roth spots, and rheumatoid factor

A definitive clinical diagnosis can be made based on the following:

1. 2 major criteria
2. 1 major criterion and 3 minor criteria
3. 5 minor criteria

DIAGNOSIS

- Diagnosis of IE is established based on Duke's criteria. However, confirm with the blood culture (3 blood cultures are taken because of high chances of false positivity, 1 positive culture is not sufficient to established the diagnosis, 2 positive blood cultures taken 12-hour apart or 3 positive blood culture taken 1-hour apart have sensitivity of 95%.

- Transthoracic echocardiography (TTE) is done in all patients with suspected endocarditis. If TTE is inconclusive and IE is suspected, then transesophageal echocardiography (TEE) is indicated.

- Do directly TEE when the prosthetic valve is implanted.

- A complete blood count will show an increase in neutrophils, ESR, and low complements level (due to activation of the immune system).

MANAGEMENT

- When IE is suspected, the best initial step is to draw cultures and then give empiric treatment with IV vancomycin and gentamicin when you wait for culture results.

- After starting empiric therapy, perform TTE to detect vegetation on the valves

- **If the culture grows methicillin-sensitive organism:** switch vancomycin to nafcillin combined with gentamicin because nafcillin is superior to vancomycin for treating methicillin sensitive organisms.

- **If the culture grows methicillin-resistant organism:** continue with vancomycin and gentamicin.

- **If the culture grows streptococcus or HACEK organisms:** switch vancomycin to IV ceftriaxone or penicillin combined with gentamicin.

- **Endocarditis on prosthetic valve:** add rifampin to above pharmacological management.

- With native-valve endocarditis, treatment is continued for about 4 weeks and with prosthetic valve endocarditis, it is continued for about 6 weeks.

- **In penicillin allergy:** continue vancomycin for methicillin-sensitive organism. In red man syndrome due to vancomycin side effects (seen within 1 hour of infusion) – slow down the infusion rate. Do not switch or stop vancomycin.

- In VRE (Vancomycin Resistant Enterococci): No therapy has been proven highly effective. In one small series of experiments, the combination of ampicillin and ceftriaxone was found to be useful against VRE. Often, the valve must be replaced to achieve a cure.

- Valve replacement is appropriate for pseudomonas or fungal endocarditis or if the patient continues to have fever and positive blood culture on 14th day despite of appropriate treatments.

- Other indications for valve replacement are persistent embolic events, congestive heart failure, vegetations greater than 1 cm in diameter, and valvular abscess formation. Strongest indication for valve replacement is valve or chordae tendinae rupture.

PROPHYLAXIS

Consider prophylaxis against IE in patients at higher risk:

- Presence of prosthetic heart valve
- History of endocarditis
- Cardiac transplant recipients who develop cardiac valvulopathy
- Congenital heart disease with a high-pressure gradient lesion

The following condition has lower risk, however, prophylaxis is recommended for them -

- Any procedure involving manipulation of gingival tissue or the periapical region of teeth, or perforation of the oral mucosa. Prophylaxis is not recommended for procedures such as endoscopy, colonoscopy, or bronchoscopy that do not require access to deep tissue or perforation of mucosa.

- Any procedure involving incision in the respiratory mucosa.

- Procedures on infected skin or musculoskeletal tissue including incision and drainage of an abscess

- Prevention of vascular catheter infections is an important prophylactic approach in preventing nosocomial infective endocarditis (NIE).

No prophylaxis is recommended for:

- For valvular pathologies such aortic-mitral stenosis/regurgitation.

- Patients with pacemakers or intra-cardiac defibrillators.

- Gastrointestinal or genitourinary procedures like colonoscopy.

- Coronary artery stent

Drugs indicated in prophylaxis:

Amoxicillin (for dental procedures), cephalexin (for skin procedures).

Azithromycin, clindamycin or vancomycin for penicillin allergy.

AORTIC STENOSIS

Aortic stenosis is the most common valvular disorder in elderly population

ETIOLOGY

- Degenerative calcification: age-related (strongest risk factor). It is the most common cause of aortic stenosis in elderly population > 65 years of age.

- Bicuspid aortic valve is the most common cause in young population between 30 to 50 years of age.

- William's syndrome (supravalvular aortic stenosis)

- Post-rheumatic disease

- Subvalvular stenosis on exertion occurs with hypertrophic obstructive cardiomyopathy (HOCM)

PATHOGENESIS

- Age-related aortic stenosis will have calcified valve that are difficult to open during systole. Endothelial cell damage due to mechanical stress occurs during the lifetime of an individual. These result in inflammation and calcification of valve.

- Chronic obstruction of left ventricular outflow will lead to left ventricular hypertrophy. In the beginning, cardiac output is normal but it decreases when severity of stenosis increases.

- Rheumatic aortic stenosis will have fusion of cusp leading to narrowed lumen across the valve.

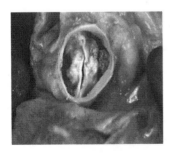
Figure 6.33: bicuspid aortic stenosis*

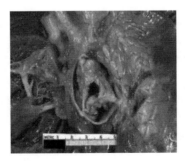
Figure 6.34: rheumatic aortic stenosis*

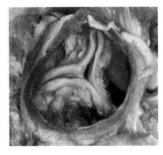
Figure 6.35: age-related aortic stenosis*

CLINICAL PRESENTATION

- Patient typically presents with shortness of breath, slow carotid upstroke, narrow pulse pressure, angina-like chest pain and syncope with exercise.

- On auscultation: crescendo-decrescendo systolic ejection murmur that radiates to carotid and right sternal border, soft or absent S2 heart sound and S4 sound is present due to left ventricular hypertrophy.

- All of the above findings develops when aortic valve orifice is less than 1 cm in diameter.

DIAGNOSIS

- Transthoracic echocardiography is best for aortic lesions.
- ECG
- Chest x-ray is done to assess the presence or absence of pulmonary congestion and other lung pathology.

- Schistiocytes can be present on peripheral smear

MANAGEMENT

- If asymptomatic then observe the patient is the general rule. Reschedule for echocardiography after 1 year.
- If symptomatic then valve replacement is the best therapy.

Recommendations for valve replacement:

- Angiography must be done before valve replacement because many times acute coronary syndrome is associated with AS. This will help to determine whether the patient is really in need of replacement or not.

- Aortic velocity greater than 4.0 m/sec or mean pressure gradient 40mmHg or higher **(even in the patient is asymptomatic if ejection fraction is < 50%).**

- Resting valve area < 1 square cm or less

- Symptoms of heart failure, ejection fraction < 50%, syncope, exertional dyspnea, angina, or pre-syncope by history or on exercise testing.

- Surgical aortic valve replacement is the preferred method for valve replacement. Less invasive procedure such as TAVR (Transcatheter Aortic Valve Replacement) is indicated when patients are at high risk or too sick for open heart surgery and predicted post TAVR survival > 12 months.

- Balloon valvuloplasty as like TAVR is limited to patients with critical aortic stenosis who are not fit for valve replacement. It is not much effective like mitral stenosis because in aortic stenosis; the problem is calcification of valve.

- Medical therapy will be ineffective, however, they can be used to manage the complication that arises due to stenosis like CHF. Caution should be taken while administering diuretics (avoid excessive diuresis) or beta-blockers.

- ACE- inhibitors, nitroglycerin, and vasodilators are absolutely contraindicated due to the risk of profound hypotension.

THUNDERNOTE: HEYDE'S SYNDROME

Heyde's syndrome is an aortic valve stenosis associated with gastrointestinal bleeding from colonic angiodysplasia.

Clinical presentation:

- Aortic stenosis with melena or hematochezia, hematemesis

Pathogenesis

- Aortic stenosis causes a form of Von-Willebrand disease by breaking down vWF which predisposed the patient to gastrointestinal bleeding.

Treatment

- Symptomatic (desmopressin) + valve replacement will cure this disease in most cases.

AORTIC REGURGITATION

In aortic regurgitation, failure of aortic valve closure during diastole leads to backflow of blood into the left ventricle.

ETIOLOGY

- Infective endocarditis
- Chronic rheumatic disease
- Aortic dissection
- Coarctation of aorta
- Tertiary syphilis
- Ankylosing spondylitis (HLA B27 serotype)

CLINICAL PRESENTATION

Acute Aortic Regurgitation

- Acute aortic regurgitation will cause sudden increase in end-diastolic value and left ventricular pressure. This will create high pressure in pulmonary circulation leading to pulmonary edema. Therefore, an acute AR presents with sudden onset of shortness of breath, chest pain if AR is associated with aortic dissection, and rapidly developing heart failure. It will not have any structural change in the heart such as eccentric hypertrophy and dilatation of left ventricle.

- On auscultation, early diastolic murmur and a soft S_1 is heard. S_1 is soft because high filling pressure in the ventricle close the mitral valve early i.e. during diastole rather than at the beginning of systole.

- Acute aortic regurgitation is a medical emergency and immediate valve replacement is required.

Chronic Aortic Regurgitation

- Patients with chronic AR often have long asymptomatic period that may last for several years. Chronic aortic insufficiency will result in cardiac remodeling. Congestive heart failure will develop over the period of time due to the volume overload.

- Patient presents with progressive shortness of breath and chest discomfort due to hyperdynamic circulation.

- Regurgitation of blood flow will cause low arterial diastolic blood pressure. Heart will pump high volume of blood into the aorta which will cause elevation of systolic blood pressure. Therefore, pulse pressure (systolic – diastolic pressure) is widened. In late stages, contractility of heart decreases resulting in low cardiac output and activation of renin-angiotensin aldosterone system ensues which will further deteriorate the patient condition by increasing afterload and volume retention.

- Physical findings that are presents in chronic aortic regurgitation includes: early diastolic murmur, Widened pulse pressure due to hyperdynamic circulation, bounding pulse (aka water-hammer pulse), bobbing and popping head with systole, and pulsation in nail beds.

DIAGNOSIS

- Transthoracic echocardiography is best for aortic lesions. If inconclusive and moderate-severe symptoms of aortic insufficiency, cardiac magnetic resonance (CMR) is indicated.
- ECG
- Chest x-ray is done to assess the presence or absence of pulmonary congestion and other lung pathology.

- In all the patients with aortic valve replacement: transesophageal echo is recommended to determine the status of the aortic valve, aorta and left ventricle.

MANAGEMENT

- In chronic asymptomatic aortic regurgitation: the aim is to decrease afterload which will increase the forward flow. It is achieved by calcium channel blockers (nifedipine) or ACE inhibitors or ARBs.

Indications for valve replacement:

- Symptomatic patient with severe aortic regurgitation regardless of left ventricular systolic function.

- Asymptomatic patients with ejection fraction less than 50%. AR patient has high ejection fraction. If the ejection fraction is below the normal level, it suggests progressive eccentric hypertrophy (remodeling) and therefore surgery is indicated to prevent these irreversible changes.

- In patients with severe AR who is undergoing cardiac surgery for other indication like CABG, mitral valve surgery or ascending aorta replacement.

- Repair the aortic sinuses or replace the ascending aorta if the left ventricular end systolic diameter is > 5.5 cm or if the diameter is > 4.5 when undergoing cardiac surgery for some other cause (e.g. in the bicuspid aortic valve).

RHEUMATIC HEART DISEASE

- Rheumatic heart disease is due to recurrent infection with Group A Streptococci in the pharynx.

- In the United States, it is more commonly seen in immigrants.

PATHOGENESIS

- During the time of infection, host develops antibodies against the M protein of group A strep. These antibodies will cross react with similar proteins found in the human tissues (type 2 hypersensitivity reaction) and lead to damage.

- Acute presentation of rheumatic heart disease occurs after 1 to 3 weeks of infection and it involve all 3 layers of heart (pancarditis). It is most common in the age group of 5 to 30 years.

- In the beginning, small thrombi develop along the lines of valve closure that do not destroy the valve (verrucous endocarditis) but with recurrent infections or untreated Strep throat, there is high risk of valvular scarring due to increase in expression of VCAM-1 which leads to infiltration of CD 4+ T cells.

- Valvular scarring will lead to commissural fusion (fish mouth deformity), thickening and fibrosis of the valve resulting in stenosis, or less commonly regurgitation.

CLINICAL PRESENTATION AND DIAGNOSIS

JONES major Criteria

- **J = Joint:** migratory polyarthritis is the most common initial presentation. Large joints such as knee, ankles and wrist are typically involved.

- **O = Heart:** pancarditis (endocarditis-myocarditis-pericarditis). It is the most common cause of death.

  In myocarditis due to rheumatic disease, Aschoff bodies (granulomatous structure consisting of fibrinoid change and lymphocytic infiltration) are pathognomonic.

  Although, Anitschkov cells (reactive histiocytes within Aschoff bodies) are associated with rheumatic heart disease, they are non-specific.

  The most common valve involved in rheumatic heart disease is the mitral valve. Aortic valve can also be affected but it will almost always have mitral valve involved. Valvular stenosis is more commonly found, however, both insufficiency and stenosis can occur together or independently.

  Severe pulmonary hypertension is a bad prognostic sign.

- **N = Nodules**: on extensor surface, the center of nodule has fibrinoid necrosis.

- **E – Erythema marginatum**: ring-shaped eruptions on the trunk or upper part of arms or legs.

- **S – Sydenham chorea**: emotional instability, muscle weakness and uncoordinated jerky movements that mainly affect the face, feet, and hands

Minor Criteria:
- Fever
- Arthralgia (pain without joint swelling)
- Increase in acute phase reactant (C-Reactive protein, ESR, neutrophils)
- Abnormal ECG

Diagnosis:
- 2 major criteria
- 1 major + 2 minor criteria
- Transthoracic echocardiography (TTE)
- If the TTE is inconclusive and there is high suspicion for mitral valve problem, then perform TEE. TEE is more sensitive and specific for mitral valve problem than TTE.

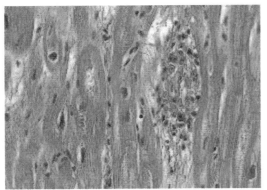
Figure 6.36: Aschoff nodule*

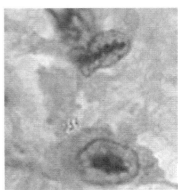
Figure 6.37: Anitskow cells*

MANAGEMENT

- Best Initial therapy in symptomatic patients: percutaneous mitral balloon commissurotomy (balloon valvuloplasty) for severe MS where mitral valve area < 1.5 square cm. Balloon valvuloplasty is contraindicated in moderate to severe mitral regurgitation and atrial thrombus.

- If balloon fails, then do valve replacement (most effective).

- Concomitant valve replacement is indicated if mitral valve area < 1.5 square cm and patient is undergoing cardiac surgery for other indications.

- If the patient is asymptomatic and stenosis is associated with atrial fibrillation, prior embolic event and left atrial thrombus: anticoagulation with **warfarin.** The goal of INR with warfarin is 2 to 3.

- If the symptoms are associated with exercise but normal sinus rhythm: heart rate control with **beta-blockers**

- If pulmonary edema is suspected: **diuretics and salt restriction**

Management for acute rheumatic heart disease:

- Primary prevention if the Strep pharyngitis is suspected in child: single IM penicillin G benzathine and 10-days of oral amoxicillin.

Secondary prophylaxis is recommended in patient with documented history of rheumatic fever or rheumatic heart disease.

- Rheumatic fever with carditis and residual valvular heart disease: antibiotic treatment for 10 years or until 40 years (whichever is longer) after the latest episode.
- Rheumatic fever with carditis but not residual valvular heart disease: antibiotic treatment for 10 years or until 21 years (whichever is longer) after the latest episode.
- Rheumatic fever without carditis: 5 years or until 21 years (whichever is longer)

Drug preferred for secondary prophylaxis: IM Penicillin G benzathine, once every 4 weeks.

MITRAL STENOSIS

Mitral stenosis is a hardening of the mitral valve, that fails to open normally during diastole. Narrowing of mitral valve orifice less than 2.5 square cm is considered to be mitral stenosis. Dilation and work hypertrophy of the left atrium will occur which predisposes to atrial fibrillation.

ETIOLOGY
- Increase in plasma volume (pregnancy)
- Rheumatic heart disease (immigrants)
- Mucopolysaccharidoses
- Endocardial fibroelastosis

CLINICAL PRESENTATION

- Mitral stenosis can be asymptomatic for long period of time. Clinical presentation become more apparent when pulmonary congestion starts developing. Pulmonary congestion will lead to pulmonary edema and hemorrhage into the alveoli. Heart failure cells can be present in sputum (rusty brown cells).

- Pulmonary congestion will produce condition similar to pulmonary stenosis which will increase the right ventricular pressure resulting in right heart failure.

- Dyspnea is the most common presentation, pulmonary rales and cough.

- Dysphagia and hoarseness due to left atrial dilation which compresses esophagus or left recurrent laryngeal nerve that is located posteriorly.

- When the structure of atria is distorted it can develop atrial fibrillation which increases the risk of systemic embolization.

PHYSICAL FINDINGS

- On auscultation, the murmur of mitral stenosis is very difficult to recognize. An opening snap followed by early to mid-diastolic rumble will be present. It is best heard at the apex of heart.

- The duration between the S2 and opening snap determines the severity of mitral stenosis. The severity of mitral stenosis increases with decrease in duration between S2 and opening snap because over the period of time, increase in right atrial pressure will cause early opening of the mitral valve and therefore, the duration between S2 and opening snap is decreased.
- Pulmonary capillary wedge pressure is high due to backward congestion. Ejection fraction will be normal because left ventricle is not affected and have lower pressure due to low volume of blood entering in the left ventricle during diastole.

DIAGNOSIS

- Transthoracic echocardiography (left atrium dilation, abnormal mitral valve movement)

- Alternative tests: transesophageal echocardiography, catheterization

- ECG is not specific but findings such as left atrial hypertrophy or atrial fibrillation can be recorded.

- Chest x-ray will show straightening of left heart border or bubble behind the heart on the lateral view.

MANAGEMENT

- Best initial therapy in symptomatic patients: percutaneous mitral balloon valvuloplasty for severe MS where mitral valve area < 1.5 square cm. Balloon valvuloplasty is contraindicated in moderate to severe mitral regurgitation and atrial thrombus.

- Balloon valvuloplasty is also indicated in asymptomatic patient with high pulmonary capillary wedge pressure (>50mmHg at rest or >60mmHg on exertion).

- If balloon fails, then do valve replacement (most effective).

- Concomitant valve replacement is indicated if mitral valve area < 1.5 square cm and patient is undergoing cardiac surgery for other indications.

- If the patient is asymptomatic and stenosis is associated with atrial fibrillation, prior embolic event and left atrial thrombus: anticoagulation with **warfarin.** The goal of INR with warfarin is 2 to 3.

- If the symptoms are associated with exercise but normal sinus rhythm: heart rate control with **beta-blockers**

- If pulmonary edema is suspected: **diuretics and salt restriction**

MITRAL STENOSIS IN PREGNANCY

- Pharmacological management should be started in symptomatic patients (3/4th patients will respond to this therapy).

- Treatment involves bed rest, oxygen therapy, and diuretics. Beta-blockers like metoprolol or atenolol is useful to prevent tachycardia and incidence of pulmonary edema during pregnancy.

- Add digoxin to beta-blockers if women develop atrial fibrillation. Do cardioversion if pharmacological managements fail to control atrial fibrillation.

- Surgery is reserved for those who deteriorate despite aggressive medical therapy.

- Anticoagulation: heparin (till 12 weeks antepartum), warfarin (12-36 weeks), heparin (36 weeks onward till delivery).

- Antibiotic prophylaxis for endocarditis is reserved only for patients with a previous history of endocarditis or presence of established infection.

- Percutaneous balloon valvuloplasty is the treatment of choice in MS associated with rheumatic heart disease. The second trimester is the preferred period for any invasive procedure.

- Surgical commissurotomy is dangerous to the fetus and last choice when valvuloplasty is contraindicated or severely calcified valve with high maternal mortality risk.

THUNDERNOTE: BALLOON VALVULOPLASTY

In balloon valvuloplasty, a balloon-tipped catheter is advanced into the left ventricle across the septum. One or two exchange guide wires are advanced through the lumen of the balloon-tipped catheter and positioned in the apex of the left ventricle or, less frequently, in the ascending aorta.

The balloon-tipped catheter is withdrawn over the guide wires, and the interatrial septum is dilated with the use of a peripheral angioplasty balloon (6-8 mm in diameter).

Finally, the balloon valvulotomy (15-20 mm in diameter) are advanced over the guide wires and positioned across the mitral valve

Contraindications:

- Mild MS

- Moderate to severe MR

- Left atrial thrombus.

The recommendation before the procedure is to perform transesophageal echocardiography to determine the presence of left atrial thrombus, with specific attention paid to the left atrial appendage.

If a thrombus is found and surgical commissurotomy is contraindicated, 3 months of anticoagulation with warfarin may result in resolution of the thrombus. Once the thrombus is resolved, perform balloon valvuloplasty.

MITRAL REGURGITATION

In mitral regurgitation, during systole, failure in proper closure of the mitral valve results in backflow of blood into the left atrium. Left ventricle will undergo eccentric hypertrophy over the period of time due to high amount of blood entering the left ventricle during diastole (regurgitated blood + venous return).

Stroke volume will be low in acute MR but it will be normal in chronic MR due to increase in left ventricular preload. Untreated mitral regurgitation will cause dilated cardiomyopathy where the stroke volume and ejection fraction are decreased and pulmonary congestion occurs.

ETIOLOGY

- Mitral valve prolapse is the most common cause of mitral regurgitation
- Posterior acute myocardial infarction (rupture of chordae tendinae)
- Dilated cardiomyopathy (stretching of mitral valve ring)
- Infective endocarditis
- Acute rheumatic fever
- SLE (lupus associated valvulopathy)

CLINICAL PRESENTATION

- Same like other valvular pathology: dyspnea (most common), pulmonary rales, cough (due to pulmonary congestion)
- Pansystolic murmur that is best heard at the apex of heart and radiates to the axilla
- S3 (in early stage) and S4 (in late stage)

DIAGNOSIS

- TTE (best initial test). If inconclusive, then do cardiac magnetic resonance (CMR).
- Cardiac catheterization is indicated when other non-invasive procedures are inconclusive.
- Before the surgery, perform transesophageal echocardiography.
- Alternative: catheterization (most accurate)

MANAGEMENT

- Vasodilator therapy is **not** indicated **in normotensive asymptomatic** patient with chronic primary mitral regurgitation and normal ejection fraction (no benefits). It is **effective for severe** acute mitral regurgitation.

- MR is a progressive disease and the onset of symptoms is the indication for surgery. Surgery must be done to prevent left heart failure.

- In asymptomatic patients, left ventricular ejection fraction <60% or left ventricular end systolic diameter > 4.0 cm is the indication for surgery.

- Normally, MR patient has normal or slightly high ejection fraction. If the ejection fraction is below the normal level, it suggests progressive eccentric hypertrophy (remodeling) and therefore surgery is indicated to prevent these irreversible changes.

- Mitral valve repair is recommended in preference to mitral valve replacement when MR is limited to posterior leaflet (if repair fails then only do surgery – mitral valve replacement)

- Cardiac resynchronization therapy along with biventricular pacing in-patient with severe MR who has conduction system abnormalities like left bundle branch block.

- If associated with infective endocarditis: antibiotics + immediate surgery

- In patients where surgery is not possible: treat with standard CHF regimen; ACE inhibitors or ARBs + beta blocker + diuretics and possibly spironolactone.

MITRAL VALVE PROLAPSE

Mitral valve prolapse is displacement of mitral valve leaflet by greater than 2mm into the left atrium during systole.

Pathogenesis: primarily due to myxomatous degeneration of the valve.

Etiology: Marfan syndrome, Ehler-Danlos syndrome, a complication of mitral regurgitation, infective endocarditis, and CHF.

Clinical presentation: often asymptomatic but can present with chest pain, palpitations, and **panic attacks**. The exact mechanism of panic attacks is unknown.

Diagnosis: TTE (best initial). If inconclusive then do TEE.

Management: beta blockers in symptomatic and tightening of the valve. Valve replacement is usually not necessary.

TRICUSPID REGURGITATION

Tricuspid regurgitation is a failure of the tricuspid valve to close properly during systole. It is mostly a feature of right heart failure and pulmonary hypertension

ETIOLOGY

- Left heart failure, inferior wall myocardial infarction, atrial fibrillation
- **Infective endocarditis (IV drug abuser)**
- Cor pulmonale: Idiopathic pulmonary hypertension (BMPR2 mutation), COPD
- **Carcinoid tumor**
- Rheumatic fever (with concomitant mitral valve association)
- Ebstein anomaly (apical displacement of the annular insertion of the septal and posterior leaflets and atrialization of a portion of the ventricular myocardium)

CLINICAL PRESENTATION

- Usually asymptomatic
- If symptomatic then symptoms of right heart failure such as hepatosplenomegaly (cardiac cirrhosis can occur), ascites, peripheral edema, and jugulovenous distension.
- Clear lungs on chest x-ray if tricuspid regurgitation is not due the left heart failure. Pulmonary findings of left heart failure will be present if tricuspid regurgitation is secondary to left side heart problems.
- Pansystolic, low-frequency murmur best heard at lower left sternal border which increases in intensity with inspiration due to increasing venous return.

DIAGNOSIS

- TTE is the best initial diagnostic test
- If inconclusive then TEE or catheterization
- CMR, ECG, chest x-ray

MANAGEMENT

- Diuretics: loops are preferred to reduce the volume overload, spironolactone
- In severe functional tricuspid regurgitation: decrease the pulmonary vascular resistance.
- Best treatment is surgery
- Tricuspid valve repair is preferred more than valve replacement

- Repair is best in functional TR due to dilation of tricuspid annular, prior evidence of left heart failure
- Replacement is best in carcinoid, radiation, Ebstein anomaly or preferred if valves are affected directly.

TRICUSPID STENOSIS

- Very rare, narrowing of the tricuspid valve orifice.
- A mid-diastolic murmur that can be heard over the left sternal border with rumbling character and tricuspid opening snap with wide splitting S1. Murmur increases in intensity with inspiration.

ETIOLOGY

- Rheumatic fever is the most common cause (almost always associated with mitral stenosis).
- Other cause can be carcinoid syndrome or congenital.

CLINICAL PRESENTATION

- The patient may complain about pulsation in the neck. Findings of right heart failure such as hepatosplenomegaly (cardiac cirrhosis can occur), ascites, peripheral edema, and jugulovenous distension [clear lungs].

- Symptoms of left heart failure will be present when associated with rheumatic fever (mitral stenosis)

DIAGNOSIS

- TTE is the best initial diagnostic test
- If inconclusive then TEE or catheterization
- CMR, ECG, chest x-ray

MANAGEMENT

- For severe-symptomatic cases: surgery is preferred over balloon valvuloplasty because most cases of severe tricuspid stenosis are accompanied with tricuspid regurgitation (rheumatic fever, carcinoid and other). Ballooning will either create or worsen tricuspid regurgitation

- Balloon valvuloplasty can be considered in isolated, symptomatic severe TS without TR.

PULMONARY STENOSIS AND REGURGITATION

- Pulmonary regurgitation is a retrograde flow of blood from the pulmonary artery to the right ventricle and pulmonary stenosis is narrowing of the pulmonary orifice.

- Pulmonary valvular pathology is least significant as compared to other because firstly it is rare and usually not severe.

- Pulmonary regurgitation can be normal in some people.

- Severe PR or PS can cause right ventricular hypertrophy and right heart failure.

ETIOLOGY

- Rheumatic fever
- Endocarditis
- Carcinoid
- Congenital (tetralogy of fallot causes PS, however, treatment of TOF later in life can result in PR, which must be surgically corrected).
- Pulmonary stenosis is usually a congenital disorder.

DIAGNOSIS

- TTE alone is usually sufficient for diagnosis and clinical decision-making.

MANAGEMENT

- Mild–moderate pulmonary regurgitation does not require any treatment or follow-up and severe pulmonary regurgitation is very uncommon.
- Treatment should focus on the primary cause of PR.
- For congenital pulmonary stenosis: balloon valvuloplasty or valve replacement.

THUNDERNOTE: PROSTHETIC VALVE

Bioprosthetic valve
- Recommended in any age group (more commonly recommended in elders > 70 years) in whom lifelong anticoagulation is not possible.

- Anticoagulation with warfarin or clopidogrel is reasonable for first 3-6 months, where the **INR should be maintained at 2.5** with warfarin therapy.

Mechanical Valve

- Recommended in patients < 60 years.

- It requires lifelong anticoagulation with warfarin, INR should be achieved at 2.5-3.0.

- Between 60 to 70 year of age: any type of valve can be used.

- Low-dose aspirin is recommended to all patients along with warfarin in mechanical valve.

Both bioprosthetic and mechanical valve are equally efficacious.

Warning
- Direct thrombin inhibitors or factor Xa inhibitors (dabigatran, rivaroxaban) are contraindicated because they cause thrombosis on mechanical valve.

- Reversal of anticoagulation in case of uncontrolled bleeding is done by fresh frozen plasma or prothrombin complex concentrate

Follow-up
- Asymptomatic uncomplicated patient is usually seen at 1 year (x-ray and ECG are not routinely indicated).
- Routine CBC and INR measurement.
- No echocardiography is indicated after postoperative evaluation (at 2-3 months) for a stable patient who does not have any discomforts i.e. no signs of valvular dysfunction.
- If the patient feels discomfort: TEE is recommended (more sensitive than TTE) for detecting prosthetic valve problems.

VALVULAR PROBLEMS BLUEPRINTS

- Transthoracic echocardiography is the best initial test. If inconclusive then do transesophageal echocardiography (more sensitive) or cardiac magnetic resonance (CMR).

- Catheterization is the most accurate test.

- Chest x-ray and ECG are non-diagnostic but are indicated in all valvular pathology for other related complications.

- Most symptoms of valvular pathology occur with exercise and therefore, exercise hemodynamics with Doppler echocardiography or cardiac catheterization can be helpful to determine exercise tolerance and severity of the disease (prognosis determination). Do not perform exercise hemodynamics if valvular problem is moderate to severe.

- Perform TEE before catheterization to rule out atrial thrombus and moderate-severe mitral regurgitation

- Valve replacement is the best therapy for aortic stenosis.

- Balloon valvuloplasty is best initial therapy for mitral stenosis. However, best is valve replacement because balloons have a high recurrence rate.

- Higher incidence in premature infants and diabetic mother
- Multifactorial inheritance (actual cause is unknown), chromosomal disorders,
- Often associated with maternal factors like smoking, alcohol, infection like rubella (PDA), drugs (lithium, vitamin A), SLE

CLINICAL PRESENTATION

- Feeding difficulty

- Sweating while feeding

- Rapid respiration

- Cyanosis

- Murmurs

- Rales on auscultation (left-sided heart failure)

- Hepatosplenomegaly (right sided heart failure)

Age is very important while assessing the child because of the difference in respiratory rate in neonates as compared to adults. They cannot complain of chest pain or shortness of breath like adults and therefore if any of the above clinical presentation is present, child requires careful evaluation.

DIAGNOSIS

- Chest x-ray is best initial test followed by other tests if required: ECG, echocardiography (best for evaluating congenital heart disease), cardiac MRI, and angiography. Many congenital heart defects can be diagnosed prenatally by fetal echocardiography.

If the baby is born with cyanotic heart disease such as transposition of great vessels and truncus arteriosus, the diagnosis is usually made shortly after birth due to cyanosis. Emergent surgery is indicated.

If the baby is born with a septal defect or an obstruction defect, often their symptoms are only noticeable after several months or sometimes even after many years.

Congenital heart diseases are broadly categorized into: cyanotic and acyanotic heart disease.

ACYANOTIC CONDITIONS

- In acyanotic condition, oxygenated blood is shunted from the left side of the heart to the right side of the heart. This oxygenated blood along with deoxygenated blood of venous return will again go through pulmonary circulation and oxygen saturation is maintained.

- 3 common types of acyanotic conditions are atrial septal defect, ventricular septal defect, and patent ductus arteriosus

CLINICAL FINDINGS: None at the birth until Eisenmenger syndrome develops.

Eisenmenger syndrome

- Shunting of blood from left to right for long period of time will cause gradual increase in right side pressure due to work hypertrophy of pulmonary vessels. When the pressure on right side is more than left side of heart, reversal of shunt will occur and some amount of deoxygenated blood will mix with oxygenated blood without undergoing pulmonary circulation.

- Patient still remain asymptomatic due enough amount of blood undergoing pulmonary circulation, however there is an increased risk of paradoxical emboli. Embolus will enter the left atrium through septal defect and then enters the systemic circulation where it can block any artery in the body.

- Cyanosis develop at late stages when the amount of deoxygenated blood passing through the septal defect is more than the amount undergoing pulmonary circulation (at low oxygen saturation).

- Patent foramen ovale is the most common septal defect present in adult (1 out of every 5 people have it). We do not treat it at birth because in most cases it will close on its own.

- Although clinical presentation is similar in various types of atrial septal defects such as ostium secundum and foramen ovale, mechanisms are different. Ostium secundum type ASD is due to an **excessive resorption** of septum primum while foramen ovale is a **residual foramen** after septum secundum covers most ostium secundum.

- Ostium secundum defect is found with mitral valve prolapse in 10-20% cases. Ostium primum defect are less common than ostium secumdum defects. Primum type defect are more commonly found in down syndrome.

- Atrial septal defects are more commonly associated with fetal alcohol syndrome, Down syndrome, and diabetic mother

DIAGNOSIS

- Child is generally diagnosed in utero by ultrasonography.
- On auscultation, wide and fixed split in S2 because an increase in blood flow across the pulmonary orifice delays closing of the pulmonary valve.
- Transthoracic echocardiography is best initial test in adults.
- Catheterization is most accurate (not detectable till 40-50 years, mostly detected in the 5th decade of life). Cardiac catherization will show increase oxygen saturation in the right atrium, right ventricle and pulmonary arteries.
- ECG shows right axis deviation (nonspecific)
- Chest x-ray

MANAGEMENT

- Asymptomatic patient does not require any treatment. When patent foramen ovale or secundum type ASD is associated with an otherwise unexplained neurologic event, traditional treatment has been antiplatelet (i.e. aspirin) therapy alone in low-risk patients or combined with warfarin in high-risk individuals to prevent cryptogenic stroke. With administration of warfarin, the international normalized ratio (INR) is maintained at 2-3.

- Surgical or percutaneous closure of the defect is preferred sometimes.

Lutembacher syndrome

- Atrial septal defect + acquired mitral stenosis
- Treated with closure of ASD and balloon valvuloplasty

Heterotaxy syndrome

- Also called as situs ambiguous, in which there is no separation between the right and left atria.

- Looks like single atrium (3 chamber heart – as like birds).

- Most organs fail to develop septum (e.g. liver or lungs), can have malrotation of the gut, biliary atresia, asplenia or polysplenia.

- Diagnosed by echocardiography, GI and liver-spleen scan, catheterization.

- Surgery is required as soon as possible depending on the severity or malformations.

Situs solitius = Normal position of organs

Situs inversus (Kartagener's syndrome) = Organs on opposite side (dextrocardia) (functional)

Situm ambigous = around the mid-line of body, can be nonfunctional.

VENTRICULAR SEPTAL DEFECT

Ventricular septal defects are collectively the most common type of congenital heart defects.

- Defect in the membranous part of interventricular septum (upper part) is most common ventricular septal defect. Less commonly, it can be present in muscular (lower part) and trabecular part of septum.

- Ventricular septal defects are usually associated with other cardiac defects such as atrial septal defect (most common), tetralogy of Fallot, patent ductus arteriosus and coarctation of aorta.

- Commonly found in fetal alcohol syndrome and diabetic mother.

- VSD can also be acquired due to rupture of septa (5-7 day after an MI)

- In endocardial cushion defect both ASD and VSD will occur along with atrioventricular valve abnormality.

DIAGNOSIS

- Child is generally diagnosed in utero by ultrasonography
- Echocardiography is best initial test
- Catheterization is most accurate. It will show an increase in PaO_2 in right ventricle and pulmonary artery. Unlike atrial septal defect, oxygen saturation is normal in the right atrium.
- Harsh pan-systolic murmur on lower left sternal border can be heard on auscultation.

MANAGEMENT

- Asymptomatic patient does not require any treatment.
- Treatment is indicated for neonates with symptomatic heart failure and moderate or large septal defect. Trial of medical therapy is recommended with furosemide and ACEi/ARBs. Digoxin is added if required. Increase in feeding is recommended.

  Many VSDs may become smaller with time and so surgery is not best initial management for acyanotic conditions. If symptoms are not controlled, schedule for surgery.

- Uncontrolled CHF with growth failure and recurrent respiratory infection is an indication for surgical repair. Neither the age nor the size of the patient is prohibitive in considering surgery.

- Large, asymptomatic defects associated with elevated pulmonary artery pressure >50mmHg are often repaired when infants are younger than 1 year, typically around the age 6 months.

- Prolapse of an aortic valve cusp is an indication for surgery even if the VSD is small. Early repair may prevent progression of the aortic insufficiency.

- Elevated pulmonary resistance despite therapy directed at the VSD may represent a primary disease of the pulmonary vessels.

PATENT DUCTUS ARTERIOSUS

- PDA is a failure of closure of ductus arteriosus after birth. Ductus arteriosus generally closes in a couple of days and its remnant in adults is called as ligamentum arteriosus. Girls are more commonly affected than boys.

- PDA is beneficial if newborn will have transposition of great vessels or other cyanotic heart disease.

- It is more commonly associated with prematurity, respiratory distress syndrome (due to persistent decrease in PaO2), down syndrome and congenital rubella (coarctation of aorta is more common).

CLINICAL PRESENTATION

- PDA is usually asymptomatic initially. However, some infants may present with rapid breathing, poor feeding habits, rapid pulse, shortness of breath, sweating while feeding, and poor growth [these findings can be present in any acyanotic condition].
- When Eisenmenger's syndrome develops, reversal of shunt will cause lower extremity cyanosis and normal upper body because of the location of ductus arteriosus (also called as differential cyanosis)

DIAGNOSIS

- Echocardiogram
- Machinery murmur is heard continuously during systolic and diastole.
- Cardiac catherization will show an increase in oxygen saturation in pulmonary arteries and normal oxygen saturation in right atrium and right ventricle.

MANAGEMENT

- Indomethacin is best initial treatment to close patent ductus arteriosus. If indomethacin fails to close ductus arteriosus and child is symptomatic, then do surgical closure.

- In certain cyanotic heart disease such as transposition of great vessels, ductus arteriosus is kept open with Prostaglandin E2.

THUNDERNOTE: Infants of Diabetic Mother

- Diabetes mellitus type 2 in more common in obese female and familial history of diabetes. Such woman generally has high level of circulating insulin level due to insulin resistance. These high levels of insulin in mother during pregnancy will diffuse across the transplacental movement into fetal circulation leading to fetal hyperinsulinemia.

- Sudden separation of the placenta during delivery will cause hypoglycemia in infant because of hyperinsulinemia in infant.

Congenital heart disease that are commonly associated in infants of diabetic mother are:

- Atrial septal defect

- Ventricular septal defect

- Patent ductus arteriosus

- Persistent truncus arteriosus

Other findings that can be present in such infants are:

- Cardiomegaly (asymmetric septal hypertrophy)
- Macrosomia
- Hyperviscosity of blood
- Small left colon syndrome
- Caudal regression syndrome.

Management

- Good glucose control during pregnancy is essential to prevent fetal anomalies.

- Management in infants of diabetic mother is symptomatic. Treat the cardiac defects if necessary and give early frequent feeds to infant.

- IV dextrose if severe hypoglycemia or if the infant does not resolve back to euglycemia.

CYANOTIC CONDITIONS

Cyanosis occurs when deoxygenated blood (low oxygen saturation) is delivered systematically without undergoing pulmonary circulation. It is more commonly seen a child whose mother has diabetes, alcoholic, malnourished, >40 years of age and had some viral infection during pregnancy.

CLINICAL PRESENTATION

- Depends on the oxygen saturation of blood
- Increase in hematocrit (polycythemia)
- Early cyanosis, syncope, clubbing of fingers (due to persistent low oxygen saturation)
- Increase risk of systemic micro emboli and endocarditis
- Surgery is required as soon as possible.

Cyanotic conditions:

- Tetralogy of fallot (TOF)
- Transposition of great vessels (TOGV)
- Total anomalous pulmonary venous return (TAPVR)
- Truncus arteriosus
- Tricuspid atresia.

TETRALOGY OF FALLOT

- TOF is the most common cause of cyanotic heart disease. Suspect TOF in a child who become cyanotic at 4-6 years of age and has tet spells.

- It is associated with chromosome 22 deletion and DiGeorge's syndrome and results from anterior mal-alignment of aorticopulmonary septum. Septum develop slightly on the right side resulting in narrowing of pulmonary artery and wide aorta that overlaps with right ventricular cavity.

- Tet spells are hypoxic spells that are characterized by transient cyanosis and rarely syncope due to sudden increase in hypoxemia under various situations like fever, hypotension, crying, anemia or events that require an increase in cardiac output. Spells can be relieved by squatting and are treated with beta-blockers like propranolol or oxygen, however, definitive cure is surgery.

Tetralogy of Fallot is characterized by:

- **Pulmonary infundibular stenosis:** determines severity and clinical presentation of TOF. If stenosis is minimal than patient will have mild symptoms or asymptomatic and if the degree of stenosis is more, than child can present with early cyanosis. Cyanosis is generally not present at the birth.

- **Ventricular septal defect:** allow mixing of oxygenated and deoxygenated blood.

- **Overriding aorta**: part of aorta begins in the right ventricle and some part in the left ventricle. Deoxygenated blood can pass through aorta from right ventricle if pulmonary stenosis is severe.

- **Right ventricular hypertrophy:** develops later on due to high stress. Hypertrophy of right ventricle will cause boot shaped appearance of heart on chest x-ray.

Diagnosis: Echocardiography is best initial investigation of choice for all congenital heart disease and surgery (timing depends on severity and child condition) is the definitive cure for most of them. Some of these children will actually require extracorporeal life support prior to surgery because of their marked hemodynamic instability.

THUNDERNOTE

VACTERL syndrome

V – Vertebral defects: hypoplastic vertebrae, risk of scoliosis

A – Anal defects: imperforated anus, do surgical repair

C – Cardiac defects: VSD > ASD > TOF

TE – Tracheoesophageal fistula: esophageal atresia with distal tracheoesophageal fistula is the most common.

R – Renal defects: incomplete formation of 1 or both kidney which causes obstruction of urine outflow or severe reflux of urine into the kidney from bladder. If uncorrected, it can lead to renal failure and may require renal transplant in early life

L – Limb defects: hypoplastic thumb, polydactyly, syndactyly, radial aplasia

Babies are born small and has difficulty in gaining weight. Development and intelligence are good.

Seen more frequently in infants born to diabetic mothers.

TRANSPOSITION OF GREAT VESSELS

TGV is a group of congenital heart defects involving an abnormal spatial arrangement of any great vessels such as superior and/or inferior vena cava (SVC, IVC), pulmonary artery, pulmonary veins, and aorta.

Congenital heart disease involving only the primary arteries (pulmonary artery and aorta) belong to a sub-group called transposition of the great arteries (TGA). It is due to a defect in spiral rotation of aorticopulmonary septum.

TOGV is the most common cause of cyanosis in an 1-day old infant.

Dextro-transposition of the great arteries

- The aorta and pulmonary artery are transposed. An aorta arises from the right ventricle and pulmonary artery arise from the left ventricle.
- Ventricles are not transposed.
- Shunts like ASD, VSD, or PDA are almost always present. Without them it would be fatal.

Levo-transposition of the great arteries

- Commonly referred to as congenitally corrected transposition of the great arteries.
- Levo-transposition is an **acyanotic CHD** in which the aorta and the pulmonary artery are transposed along with the left and right ventricles.

TRICUSPID ATRESIA

There is a complete absence of the tricuspid valve or no outlet from the right atrium to the right ventricle. This will also result in the absence of right atrioventricular connection.

Both ASD and VSD are necessary for survival. hypoplastic right ventricle.

- The patient might have holosystolic murmur along the left sternal border depending upon the VSD size. Another finding that is present in tricuspid atresia is single second heart sound due absence of right sided flow into the right ventricle and hypoplastic right ventricle.

- ECG will show left axis deviation plus left ventricular hypertrophy.

- Echocardiogram is best initial diagnostic test.

- **Management:** Prostaglandin E1 to keep the patent ductus arteriosus open is best initial step in management followed by atrial balloon septostomy to allow blood circulation. Surgical repair is done after that.

  The ductus arteriosus is kept open till surgical repair because some amount of blood will regurgitate back through it and undergo oxygenation via pulmonary circulation. If the child is hemodynamically unstable, extracorporeal life support is also required prior to surgery.

PERSISTENT TRUNCUS ARTERIOSUS

- Truncus arteriosus fails to properly divide into the pulmonary trunk and aorta due to the failure in development of aorticopulmonary septum.
- Mixed venous and arterial blood is delivered to the pulmonary and systemic circulation.

TOTAL ANOMALOUS PULMONARY VENOUS RETURN (TAPVR)

- Pulmonary veins do not connect normally to the left atrium; instead, they drain abnormally in the right atrium (cardiac TAPVR) or superior vena cava (supracardiac TAPVR) or inferior vena cava (infracardiac TAPVR).

- ASD or VSD or PDA are necessary for survival till surgery is done. It is managed similarly to other cyanotic heart disease – Keep PDA open and extracorporeal life support prior to surgery.

- There will be right ventricular overflow and left sided hypoplasia.

HYPOPLASTIC HEART SYNDROME

- Hypoplasia can affect the heart, typically resulting in the underdevelopment of the right ventricle or the left ventricle.

- It is rare but is the most serious form of congenital heart disease

- Hypoplastic left heart syndrome can be seen in total anomalous pulmonary venous return and hypoplastic right heart syndrome can be seen in tricuspid atresia. Hypoplastic heart syndrome can also be idiopathic without any underlying abnormality.

- In both conditions, the presence of a patent ductus arteriosus and patent foramen ovale are essential for the infant to survive until emergency heart surgery can be performed.

Aorticopulmonary Septum Anomalies	
Tetralogy of fallot	Right shift of septum
Transposition of great arteries	Failure in the spiralization of septum
Persistent truncus arteriosus	Failure in the formation of septum

VALVULAR DEFECTS

Pulmonary stenosis (infundibular)

- Pulmonary stenosis is most common valvular congenital heart disease that is associated with tetralogy of Fallot. It creates dynamic or fixed obstruction to flow from the right ventricle of the heart to the pulmonary artery.

- Valves are usually normal; stenosis is due to constriction of pulmonary artery.

- Echocardiography shows post-stenotic dilation of the pulmonary artery and ECG will show right ventricular and atrial hypertrophy.

Ebstein's anomaly

- Septal leaflet of the tricuspid valve is displaced towards the apex of right ventricle of the heart.
- Ebstein's anomaly is more commonly found in woman with bipolar disorder who is taking lithium during the 1st trimester.
- It is also rarely associated with Wolf Parkinson White syndrome.

Pulmonary atresia

- Malformation of the pulmonary valve in which the valve orifice fails to develop.
- The valve is completely closed thereby obstructing the outflow of blood from the heart to the lungs.

Bicuspid aortic valve

- Two of the three aortic valve leaflets fuse during the development resulting in a bicuspid valve instead of a normal tricuspid configuration.
- Biscuspid aortic valve is the most common cardiac anomaly that can be seen in Turner's syndrome. Turner syndrome can also develop coarctation of aorta and mitral valve prolapse. Coarctation of aorta in newborn is generally fatal.

- Congenital coronary artery abnormalities are very rare and sometimes can be **benign** like myocardial bridges.

- **Myocardial bridge:** Coronary artery passes through the myocardium instead of resting on top of it. Constriction of artery occurs during systole. It is very common and found in 1% population. Less than 50% blockage is considered benign and will variable manifestations. No treatment is indicated for benign condition.

- **Anomalous origin of left coronary artery arising from the pulmonary artery (ALCAPA):** rare, usually isolated cardiac anomaly due to persistence of pulmonary buds and involution of aortic buds. Pulmonary buds will form the coronary arteries or abnormal conotruncal septation.

- Clinical manifestations depends on the severity of anomaly. Severe anomalies can present in infancy while mild anomalies can present in adults or sometimes remain asymptomatic throughout life.

CLASSIFICATION

- **Anomalies of origination and course**: anomalous location of coronary ostium, single coronary artery.

- **Anomalies of intrinsic coronary arterial anatomy:** congenital ostial stenosis or atresia, coronary ectasia or an aneurysm.

- **Anomalies of coronary termination**: fistulas from coronary artery to other non-cardiac vessels or organs, inadequate arteriolar/capillary branching.

BEST DIAGNOSTIC TEST: Angiography

MANAGEMENT

- In symptomatic patient (presentation of congestive heart failure or ischemic heart disease): medical treatment, coronary angioplasty with stent deployment, and surgical repair. Due to limited data, manifestations and pathophysiological mechanisms are highly variable.

CONGENITAL PROLONG QT SYNDROME

- **Jervell and Lange-Nielsen syndrome:** autosomal recessive **defect in potassium channels**, prolonged QT on ECG + congenital deafness.

- **Romano-Ward syndrome**: autosomal dominant, defect in potassium channels, Prolonged QT not associated with deafness.

  Prolong QT occurs due to an abnormal repolarization of the heart, which causes a difference in the refractory period of heart muscle cells. 2.5% of population have prolonged QT interval and thus diagnose is given after following "LQTS diagnostic score"

- Electrolyte imbalance and drugs can also cause QT prolongation

- Prolong QT syndrome have high risk of re-entrant ventricular arrhythmias such as torsades de pointes.

DOUBLE INLET LEFT VENTRICLE

- Both the left atrium and the right atrium drain into the left ventricle.
- The right ventricle is hypoplastic or doesn't exist

DOUBLE OUTLET RIGHT VENTRICLE

- Both of the great arteries connect (in whole or in part) to the right ventricle.
- In some cases, this occurs on the left side of the heart rather than the right side.

INTERRUPTED AORTIC ARCH

- Very rare, the aorta is not completely developed. There is a gap between the ascending and descending thoracic aorta which is also called as complete form of a coarctation of the aorta.
- Interrupted aortic arch is associated with DiGeorge syndrome

PENTALOGY OF CANTRELL

It involves the diaphragm, abdominal wall, pericardium, heart and lower sternum.

- Omphalocele
- Anterior diaphragmatic hernia
- Sternal cleft
- Ectopia Cordis
- Intracardiac defect: either VSD or a diverticulum of the left ventricle.

SHONE'S ANOMALY

Shone's anomaly is the set of **four left-sided cardiac defects:**

- Supravalvular mitral membrane
- Mitral valve prolapse
- Subaortic stenosis (membranous or muscular)
- Coarctation of the aorta

ECTOPIA CORDIS

- The heart is abnormally located either partially or completely outside the thorax.
- Very rare and very high mortality
- It is usually associated with other congenital heart diseases and non-cardiac problems such as omphalocele, and cleft palate.

NARROW QRS COMPLEX

Narrow QRS complex is almost always due to supraventricular arrhythmia. Supraventricular tachycardia originates from the location within the heart above the bundle of His. Patients are generally asymptomatic but can present with palpitations, fatigue, light-headedness, chest discomfort, dyspnea and rarely syncope.

Sinus Tachycardia:

- Sinus tachycardia is non-paroxysmal (starts and end gradually). It is defined as heart rate greater than 100bpm. ECG will show regular rhythm, normal P wave and PR interval and QRS complex < 0.12 seconds. It requires evaluation of stressors such infection or volume depletion.

Paroxysmal Supraventricular Tachycardia:

- Paroxysmal supraventricular tachycardia (PSVT) are episodes of regular and paroxysmal palpitations with sudden onset and termination. If the termination is by vagal maneuvers it is suggestive of atrioventricular re-entrant tachycardia (AVRT).

Atrioventricular Nodal Reentrant Tachycardia:

- It occurs when re-entrant pathway forms within or just next to AV node. In AVNRT, the fast and slow pathways are **located within the right atrium** close to or within the AV node and **have electrophysiological property like AV node.** Therefore, an episode of AVNRT can be terminated by any action that blocks the AV node such as vagal maneuver and beta blockers.

- Unlike AVRT, there is no accessory connection between atrium and ventricles. P wave can be hidden behind the QRS complex or occur after QRS complex.

- After diagnosing AVNRT by ECG and adenosine test, electrophysiological studies are done for confirmation. If the patient is hemodynamically unstable, catheter ablation of slow pathway can potentially cure AVNRT.

Atrioventricular Reentrant Tachycardia:

- It occurs when accessory pathway is located between the atria and ventricles. A classic example is Wolf-Parkinson-White syndrome. During AVRT, electrical signal passes in the normal manner from the AV node into the ventricles. It then, pathologically, passes back into the atria via the accessory pathway causing atrial contraction and returns to the AV node. Once initiated, the cycle may continue causing an episode of tachycardia.

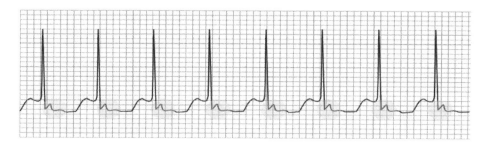

Figure 8.1: Atrioventricular nodal re-entrant tachycardia*

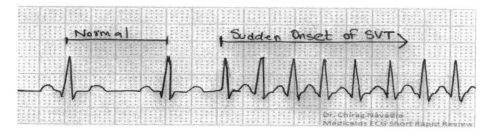

Figure 8.2: paroxysmal supraventricular tachycardia

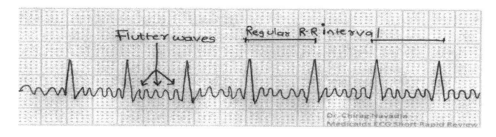

Figure 8.3: atrial flutter

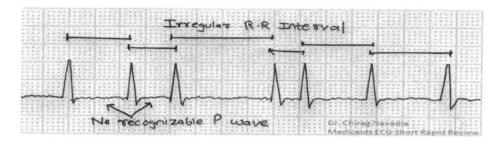

Figure 8.4: atrial fibrillation

DIAGNOSIS

Evaluation of ECG with narrow QRS complex (<120ms):

- If irregular tachycardia: atrial fibrillation, multifocal atrial tachycardia
- If regular rhythm and P wave not visible: AVNRT
- If regular rhythm, P wave visible and atrial rate is greater than ventricular rate: Atrial flutter or atrial tachycardia
- If regular rhythm, P wave visible but atrial rate is not greater than ventricular rate, check RP interval. If RP interval longer than PR interval: Atrial tachycardia, PJRT, atypical AVNRT. If RP interval shorter than PR interval: AVRT (>70ms), atrial tachycardia and AVNRT (<70 ms).

Effects of Adenosine administration:

- **No change in rate**: Dose is not enough or ventricular tachycardia

- **Sudden termination of narrow complex:** AVNRT (Atrioventricular Nodal Reentrant Tachycardia), AVRT (Atrioventricular Reentrant Tachycardia) (Ablate the reentrant pathway later on)

- **Gradual slowing and then again narrow QRS**: sinus tachycardia, nonparoxysmal junctional tachycardia.

- **Persistent narrow QRS but develops AV block:** Atrial flutter or Atrial tachycardia

Other diagnostic tests that are indicated:

- 24-hour Holter monitoring can be use in people with frequent but transient arrhythmias

- Exercise testing is less useful unless arrhythmias are triggered by exertion.

- Use electrophysiological ablation for diagnosis and therapy in cases with clear history of paroxysmal regular palpitations.

  Before referring to electrophysiological studies, if the patient has symptoms but ECG is inconclusive: evaluate for other causes like hyperthyroidism, drugs, nicotine, and alcohol intake.

- Echocardiography is ordered to exclude other structural heart defects.

- Atrial fibrillation can occur secondary to hypertension, hyperthyroidism, cocaine, dilated cardiomyopathy, valvular heart disease, and pericarditis. Rule out all possible etiology.

MANAGEMENT

- Narrow QRS with normal ECG (sinus rhythm, no pre-excitations) and normal left ventricular function requires no treatment.

Management of PSVT and AVRNT in hemodynamically stable patient:

- Vagal maneuver is best initial management for PSVT and AVNRT.

- If fails to control, then give IV adenosine (blocks atrioventricular node). Adenosine should be avoided in patients with severe bronchial asthma. Its effects are potentiated by dipyridamole. Be careful if the patient is on dipyridamole.

- Do rate control with IV verapamil/diltiazem/beta blocker. Procainamide is indicated for WPW syndrome (more details are discussed in next chapter). In AVRT, avoid anything that blocks AV node.

Management of atrial fibrillation/flutter in hemodynamically stable patient:

- The aim is to prevent ventricular arrhythmia. This is primarily achieved by rate and rhythm control.

- Medications that are used for rate control is IV verapamil or diltiazem or beta blockers. [immediate cardioversion for unstable patient].

- After rate control, if atrial fibrillation persists or patient develops AV block; rhythm control with pharmacological or electrical cardioversion is indicated. Pharmacological cardioversion can be achieved by IV dofetilide or IV amiodarone.

- Before doing elective cardioversion in a stable patient, perform **transesophageal** echocardiography to check for the mural thrombus. Mural thrombus can develop if atrial fibrillation is present for more than 48 hours. If the mural thrombus is present, then start warfarin and heparin to avoid a stroke. Warfarin is generally continued for 3 weeks prior to cardioversion.

- Rate control along with anticoagulation is superior to rhythm control in hemodynamically stable patient and therefore; rate control is attempted before rhythm control.

- Give oxygen to every patient with atrial fibrillation even if oxygen saturation is normal. Elective cardioversion is still an option if patient does not want to take medications.

Management of atrial fibrillation with decompensated heart failure:

- Add digoxin (mild rate control + increase inotropy will improve ejection fraction) to standard treatment of decompensated heart failure.

- Amiodarone or dofetilide can be given only if symptoms persist with low ejection fraction.

Management of atrial fibrillation with structural heart disease or low ejection fraction:

- Amiodarone is superior to other drugs.

Management of atrial fibrillation in hemodynamically unstable patient:

- Immediate cardioversion is required. No airway, no breathing should be tried first (waste of time).

  Unstable patient means - hypotension or shortness of breath or altered mental status or angina-type chest pain. Any 1 of this 4 is enough to label patient as unstable.

Long term management of atrial fibrillation:

After the rate or rhythm control, start anticoagulation therapy for 4 to 6 weeks depending upon CHADS2 score and send the patient home with metaprolol (+/- digoxin +/- diuretics) and anticoagulant.

CHAD-S2 score is used to estimate the risk of stroke in patients with non-rheumatic atrial fibrillation. A high CHADS$_2$ score corresponds to a greater risk of stroke while a low CHADS$_2$ score corresponds to a lower risk of stroke.

CHAD-S2 SCORE	
C: Congestive heart failure	1
H: Hypertension: blood pressure consistently > 140/90 mmHg after (or treated HT on medication), hyperthyroidism	1
A: Age older than 75 years	1
D: Diabetes mellitus	1
S2: Prior stroke or transient ischemic attack	2

Score 0 = Low risk = Daily baby aspirin (81mg)

Score 1 = Moderate risk = Aspirin or warfarin at INR 2.0-3.0, Rivaroxaban or dabigatran (more effective than warfarin but no antidote, high risk of renal failure and GI bleeding)

Score 2 = High risk = Warfarin at INR 2.0-3.0, Rivaroxaban (factor X inhibitor) or dabigatran (direct thrombin inhibitor).

THUNDERNOTE: AndeXanet

(This is neither a drug promotion nor will be tested on USMLE till FDA approval)

Andexanet may become first FDA approved antidote for factor Xa inhibitor. After its approval, I personally believe that Factor Xa drugs will essentially replace warfarin almost everywhere with few exceptions and contraindications such as GI bleeding and renal failure. Andexanet has recently passed phase 3 clinical trials **(December, 2015).**

- Wide QRS complex means QRS duration > 120 msec.

- Unlike narrow complex tachycardia (always supraventricular), Wide QRS does not mean that the problem is always ventricular. It can be either supraventricular or ventricular.

VENTRICULAR TACHYCARDIA

- Ventricular tachycardia refers to any rhythm faster than 100 beats per minute, with 3 or more irregular beats in a row, arising distal to the bundle of His.
- No P wave is noticeable (hidden behind the complex)
- Multiple ectopic irritable foci (ischemia, digoxin, electrolyte imbalance, dilated cardiomyopathy) or re-entrant phenomenon will cause ventricular tachycardia.
- Ventricular tachycardia may complicate into life threatening ventricular fibrillation and sudden cardiac death.

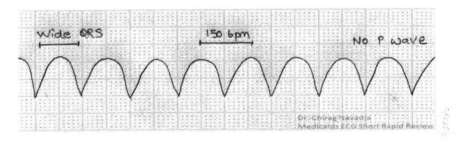

Figure 8.5: ventricular tachycardia (monomorphic)

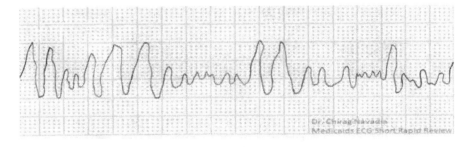

Figure 8.6: ventricular fibrillation

- In monomorphic type: the shape, size and amplitude of QRS complex will be same.
- In polymorphic type: different types of complex are present.

DIAGNOSIS

Evaluation of ECG with wide QRS complex (>120msec)

- If the rhythm is irregular, then diagnose can be atrial fibrillation/flutter/tachycardia **with variable conduction and bundle branch block.**

- If the rhythm is regular or ventricular rate faster than atrial rate, then diagnose can be Right bundle branch block, Left bundle branch block, ventricular tachycardia.

- If distinct QRS pattern in all precordial leads with QS complex only: diagnostic for ventricular tachycardia.

Other diagnostic tests that are indicated:

- 24-hour Holter monitoring can be use in people with frequent but transient arrhythmias

- Exercise testing is less useful unless arrhythmias are triggered by exertion.

- Use electrophysiological ablation for diagnosis and therapy in cases with clear history of paroxysmal regular palpitations.

  Before referring to electrophysiological studies, if the patient has symptoms but ECG is inconclusive: evaluate for other causes like hyperthyroidism, drugs, nicotine, and alcohol intake.

- Echocardiography is ordered to exclude other structural heart defects.

THUNDERNOTE: Electrophysiological Studies

- In this method, recording and stimulating electrodes are inserted via right- or left-sided cardiac catheterization into all 4 cardiac chambers.

- Atria are paced from the right or left atrium, ventricles are paced from the right ventricular apex or right ventricular outflow tract, and cardiac conduction is recorded. Programmed stimulation techniques may be used to trigger and terminate a reentrant arrhythmia.

CARDIOVERSION vs DEFEBRILLATION

Cardioversion is a synchronized administration of shock during the R waves or QRS complex of a cardiac cycle.

Defibrillation is a nonsynchronized random administration of shock during a cardiac cycle.

It causes all of the heart cells to contract simultaneously. This interrupts and terminates abnormal electrical rhythm. This, in turn, allows the sinus node to resume normal pacemaker activity. They are contraindicated in dysrhythmias due to enhanced automaticity such as digitalis toxicity, multifocal atrial tachycardia. If performed, life threatening ventricular arrhythmias can occur.

Defibrillation and cardioversion are also ineffective in asystole because they terminate abnormal electrical rhythm and allow time for SA for resume normal activity. In asystole, there is no normal or abnormal rhythm. Perform CPR and give epinephrine.

MANAGEMENT

For hemodynamically stable patient with ventricular tachycardia:

- Procainamide or lidocaine or amiodarone are indicated

- If the patient is stable and ECG findings are nonspecific: perform adenosine test. If tachycardia is supraventricular, adenosine administration will stop them. If the origin of tachycardia is ventricular, adenosine administration won't help. One of the above antiarrhythmic is recommended.

- If antiarrhythmic fail to control arrhythmia, then perform cardioversion.

- After terminating the episodes, AICD (Automated Implantable Cardioverter Defibrillator) is indicated for long term management in hemodynamically stable patient with wide QRS complex.

- If the arrhythmia is due to acute ischemic cause give Beta-Blocker. However, if arrhythmia is not terminated, perform cardioversion.

For unstable patient with ventricular tachycardia and pulse is present:

- Best initial management is synchronized cardioversion.

For unstable patient with ventricular fibrillation or pulseless ventricular tachycardia:

- Perform unsynchronized cardioversion immediately and then do CPR.

- If the heart rhythm is not restored, besides CPR and defibrillation, **add** IV epinephrine after 2nd shock.

- If the patient continues to have ventricular fibrillation or pulseless ventricular tachycardia, **add** antiarrhythmic like procainamide or lidocaine after 3rd shock.

THUNDERNOTE: Graves' Disease

- Graves' disease is a type of primary hyperthyroidism, which presents with symptoms of palpitation, anxiety, hand tremors, weight loss, tachycardia, pretibial myxedema, and exophthalmos.

- Fibroblasts in the orbital tissues may express the TSH receptor which leads to accumulation of glycosaminoglycan behind the eyeball

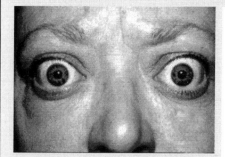

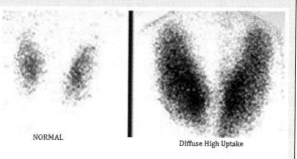

NORMAL

Diffuse High Uptake

Figure 8.7: proptosis and lid retraction*

Figure 8.8: diffuse radioactive iodine uptake

- Hyperthyroidism in Graves' disease occurs due to continuous stimulation of TSH receptors by antithyroglobulin antibodies that result in high level of circulating thyroid hormone. This high level of thyroid hormone will act negatively on the hypothalamus and decreases TSH production

- Ventricular fibrillation is the most common cause of death in Grave's disease.

- The patient is treated with beta-blockers with methimazole or propylthiouracil.

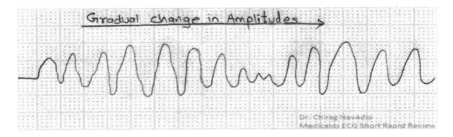

Figure 8.9: torsade-de-pointes

Torsades-De-Pointes is characterized by a gradual change in the amplitude and twisting of the QRS complexes around the isoelectric line.

This rhythm is an unusual variant of polymorphic ventricular tachycardia with the normal or long QT intervals. It may deteriorate into ventricular fibrillation or asystole.

ETIOLOGY

- Drugs (tricyclic antidepressants, macrolides, antipsychotic, methadone, antiarrhythmic, quinolones that prolong QT interval)
- Congenital long QT syndrome (defect in potassium channels)
- Electrolyte abnormalities such as hypomagnesemia

CLINICAL PRESENTATION

- Recurrent episodes of palpitations, dizziness, and syncope; however, sudden cardiac death can occur with the first episode.
- Nausea, cold sweats, shortness of breath, and chest pain also may occur but are nonspecific and can be produced by any form of tachyarrhythmia.

MANAGEMENT

For hemodynamically stable patient:

- Magnesium sulphate (decreases the influx of calcium, thus lowering the amplitude of action potentials).

- Beta-1 agonist drugs (to increase heart rate and decrease prolonged QT interval).

- If torsades convert into ventricular fibrillation (unstable): Unsynchronized cardioversion is required.

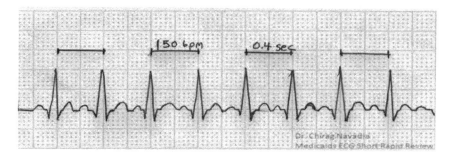

Figure 8.10: sinus tachycardia

- Sinus tachycardia is the diagnosis when the sinus rhythm is greater than 100 bpm.

- Normal P-wave (different shapes of P' wave is present in **atrial tachycardia**)

- Sinus tachycardia is not paroxysmal.

ETIOLOGY

- Occurs due to some underlying conditions such as hyperthyroidism, hypovolemia, fever, exercise and possibly due to the failure of the mechanism that controls sinus rate. Drugs (caffeine, nicotine, salbutamol, amphetamine, cocaine can also cause sinus tachycardia.

Postural orthostatic sinus tachycardia: Sinus tachycardia in upright position (standing)

Sinus node reentrant tachycardia: due to re-entry phenomenon

Inappropriate sinus tachycardia: Persistent tachycardia unrelated or out of proportion of any stress. It is due to enhanced SA node automaticity or high SNS activity.

MANAGEMENT

- Treat the underlying cause.
- In symptomatic sinus tachycardia: beta-blocker or calcium channel blocker (verapamil).

- In WPW, an accessory conduction pathway is present between atria and ventricles (a type of atrioventricular reentrant tachycardia, narrow QRS complex).

- Electrical impulses are rapidly conducted to the ventricles. These rapid impulses create a slurring of the initial portion of the QRS complex called as **Delta wave.**

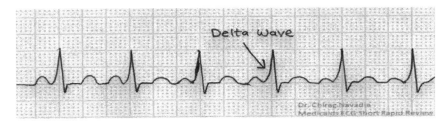

Figure 8.11: Wolf-Parkinson-White syndrome

- Patient with WPW remain asymptomatic during childhood but WPW become increasingly problematic in adult years, when atrial dilation or surgical scars predispose the patient to atrial flutter or atrial fibrillation with potential for rapid conduction over an accessory pathway.

- Loud S1 can be heard on auscultation.

- Electrophysiology studies are done to confirm the location of the conduction pathway and evaluate specific treatments. It is done before ablation.

MANAGEMENT

- **Asymptomatic patient:** not treated. Do not slow AV conduction in asymptomatic patient (avoid digoxin or calcium channel blockers in asymptomatic).

- **Asymptomatic patient with structural heart disease or shortest RR interval <250ms:** Catheter ablation

- **Symptomatic patient but hemodynamically stable:** Electrophysiological studies with ablation is best initial approach. Pharmacotherapy is also appropriate if symptoms are mild and no other structural heart disease is present. Drug of choice include: Procainamide with flecainide or sotalol with amiodarone.

- **Hemodynamically unstable patient:** Catheter ablation is the best therapy.

FOCAL JUNCTIONAL TACHYCARDIA

- Junctional tachycardia arises from AV node or bundle of his. They are very rare and pediatric patients are more commonly affected.
- Non-paroxysmal in nature.
- If presented in adulthood, it is usually benign and associated with stress or exercise or congenital septal defects.
- Junctional non-paroxysmal tachycardia can arise in digitalis toxicity, myocardial infarction or post-surgery.
- On ECG, atrioventricular dissociation is present. Heart rate of 110-250 bpm and a narrow complex or typical BBB pattern is noticeable. Sometime junctional rhythm looks like atrial fibrillation.

MANAGEMENT

- Severely symptomatic patient: ablation
- Moderately symptomatic: beta blocker or flecainide
- If mild or asymptomatic: manage the underlying cause

MULTIFOCAL ATRIAL TACHYCARDIA

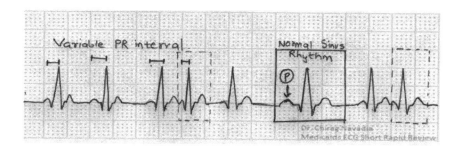

figure 8.12: multifocal atrial tachycardia

- Irregular tachycardia with 3 or more different 'P' wave morphology. P' wave is determined by the location of focus in atrium.
- It is usually associated with pulmonary disease such as COPD. Rarely, it is associated with electrolyte abnormalities due to digoxin excess.
- Treat the underlying condition.
- Calcium channel blockers can be use but less effective.
- The main point is - avoid beta-blockers.

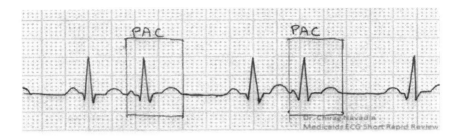

Figure 8.13: premature atrial contractions

- Premature atrial contractions are common in pregnancy (50% cases). They are benign findings and generally well tolerated

- It occurs when another region of the atria depolarizes before the sinoatrial node and triggers a premature heartbeat.

- On ECG, a single whole complex occurs earlier than the next expected sinus complex. Sinus rhythm usually resumes after PAC.

- Symptomatic exacerbation of supraventricular tachycardia can occur rarely (0.1% case).

As all antiarrhythmic drugs crosses placenta, treatment of supraventricular tachycardia is a major concern for the fetus (fetal growth and proarrhythmic).

- All drugs are class C except sotalol and amiodarone (class B) or atenolol (class D).

- No drug is recommended if the patient has mild symptoms. Reassure the patient.

- Drugs are recommended only if the symptoms are intolerable or hemodynamic compromise.

- Catheter ablation is the procedure of choice in drug-refractory cases (if needed, do it in 2nd trimester)

PREMATURE VENTRICULAR CONTRACTIONS

Premature ventricular contractions are intermittent arrhythmia with wide QRS complex of bizarre morphology, and compensatory pause. PVCs may occur singly, in clusters of two or more, or in repeating patterns, such as bigeminy or trigeminy.

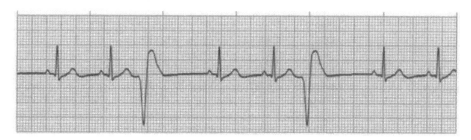

Figure 8.13.2: premature ventricular contraction (trigeminy)*

ETIOLOGY

- PVCs can be seen in normal individuals, but are more common in patients with underlying cardiac pathology such as myocardial infarction or electrolyte abnormalities.
- PVCs are usually caused by electrical irritability in the ventricular conduction system or muscle tissue. This irritability may be provoked by anything that disrupts normal electrolyte shifts during cell depolarization and repolarization.

MANAGEMENT

There are no specific antiarrhythmic medications that has shown to improve survival.

- If the patient is asymptomatic: no treatment
- If the patient is symptomatic: beta-blockers is drug of choice. Amiodarone is second-line therapy for symptomatic PVCs.

THUNDERNOTE: HYPERKALEMIA

- Hyperkalemia is defined as potassium level > 5.0 mEq/l (normal is 3.5 to 5.0 mEq/l). Level above 6.5 mEq/l is a medical emergency.

ETIOLOGY

- Acute trauma (release of potassium from cell rupture)

- Impairment in potassium excretion (chronic renal disease)

- Medications (ACE inhibitors/ARBs, NSAIDs, potassium-sparing diuretics, digoxin, statins + gemfibrozil and others)

- Addison's disease, congenital adrenal hyperplasia (21-hydroxylase deficiency), Type 4 renal tubular acidosis, diabetes mellitus type 1 (low insulin).

- Consuming high potassium diet will not cause hyperkalemia unless kidney function is compromised.

CLINICAL PRESENTATION

- Mild to moderate hyperkalemia are usually asymptomatic

- Neurological symptoms are rarely present such as general weakness, flaccid paralysis, abdominal pain, and myalgia

- ECG changes will show peaked T-wave, PR prolongation and QRS widening.

MANAGEMENT

- Start immediate management if the patient is symptomatic and ECG is abnormal.

- Combination of calcium gluconate, insulin and glucose is best initial step in management of hyperkalemia. Calcium gluconate will stabilize cardiac membrane and prevent life threatening arrhythmias and Insulin will push potassium and glucose into the cell lowering the circulating free potassium.

- Polystyrene sulphate (kayexalete) is used for long-term management if necessary. It binds potassium in the gastrointestinal tract and prevent absorption. Kayexalate neither decrease the effect of high potassium on cardiac muscle nor it lowers potassium level acutely.

- Rule out and treat the underlying cause later.

- Withdrawal of offending agent if potassium level > 6.0 mEq/l. Do not start on digoxin or ACE inhibitors if potassium level is greater than 5.0 mEq/l.

- Beta 2 agonist (nebulized albuterol)

- Diuretics (furosemide, thiazides) can be used for long-term management if necessary.

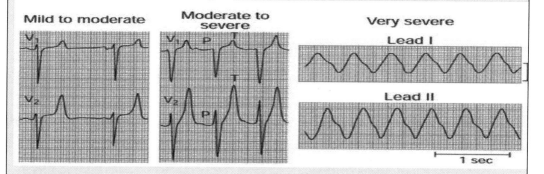

Figure 8.14: peak T-wave that will eventually lead to ventricular tachycardia*

Cardiac medications that cause hyperkalemia:

- Nonselective beta blockers: interfere with beta-2 mediated intracellular potassium uptake.

- ACE inhibitors: inhibition of angiotensin II formation with a subsequent decrease in aldosterone secretion. Aldosterone gets rid of potassium in exchange of sodium.

- ARBs: blocks angiotensin I receptor and decreases aldosterone secretion.

- K+ sparing diuretics: blocks epithelial sodium channel or aldosterone receptors.

- Cardiac glycosides (digoxin): inhibits Na-K-ATPase pump and therefore potassium cannot go inside the cell.

FIRST DEGREE AV BLOCK

First-degree heart block is the prolongation of the PR interval >200 msec. First-degree AV block occurs when impulses from the atria are consistently delayed when passing through the AV node. Conduction eventually occurs, it just takes longer than normal. The area of delay is almost always located above the AV node (supranodal).

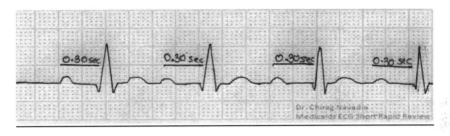

Figure 8.15: prolonged PR interval (first degree heart block)

CLINICAL PRESENTATION

The patient is usually asymptomatic and first degree AV block is an incidental finding on the ECG.

It is a physiological finding in healthy individuals with high vagal tone (athletes). Although symptoms are rare in idiopathic first degree AV block, they may result from transient high-degree AV block associated with other cardiac conditions or medications.

No other diagnostic or laboratory test is indicated for first degree AV block and Mobitz type 1 AV block.

ETIOLOGY (same for all heart blocks)

Temporary block: inferior wall MI, digoxin toxicity, beta blockers, calcium blockers and cardiac surgery.

Permanent block: aging, congenital abnormalities (SLE), anteroseptal MI, cardiomyopathy, and cardiac surgery.

MANAGEMENT

- **If the patient is asymptomatic:** no treatment
- **If the patient is symptomatic:** atropine is the drug of choice
- Long term therapy is generally not indicated.

SECOND DEGREE AV BLOCK (MOBITZ TYPE 1)

Mobitz type 1 AV block has gradual prolongation of PR interval followed by drop beat. Type 1 AV blocks are almost always located in the AV node and will have narrow QRS complex.

Ischemia involving right coronary artery is one of the many potential cause. Right coronary artery supplies AV node in 80% of population and obstruction will cause ischemic change in AV node. In 20% of population, AV node is supplied by left coronary artery.

Ratio of P waves to QRS complex is 2:1, or 3:2, or 4:3. It is the number of P' wave and QRS complex after which a drop beat occurs.

- 3:2 ratio means, 3 P' waves and 2 QRS complex are present before every drop beat.
- 4:3 ratio means, 4 P' waves and 3 QRS complex are present before every drop beat. The mathematical formula to describe this ratio is X:(X-1).

Exercise testing is used to evaluate 2:1 heart block if Mobitz type 1 and Mobitz type 2 are difficult to differentiate on ECG because in Mobitz type 2, the block becomes more significant and often symptomatic which requires additional management such as 24-hour holter monitoring and electrophysiological studies.

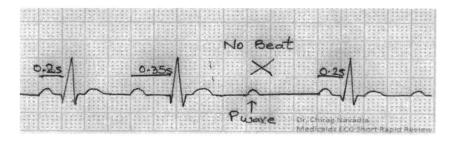

Figure 8.16: 3:2 AV block (drop beat occur after 3 P' waves and 2 QRS complex)

CLINICAL PRESENTATION

- The patient is usually asymptomatic at rest. Although rare, Mobitz type 1 AV block may reduce exercise tolerance in some patients with left ventricular systolic dysfunction associated with other cardiac conditions or medications.

MANAGEMENT

- **If the patient is asymptomatic:** no treatment
- **If the patient is symptomatic:** atropine is the drug of choice.
- Long term therapy is generally not indicated.

- Digoxin, beta-blockers and calcium channel blockers are avoided if possible because they will slower the AV conduction and increase the risk of syncope.

SECOND DEGREE AV BLOCK (MOBITZ TYPE 2)

Mobitz type 2 AV block is characterized by a **constant** prolongation of PR interval followed by an entire drop of a beat due to failure in conduction of an electrical signal to the ventricles.

Mobitz type 2 AV block is almost always located in the bundle branches and often involves both right and left bundle branches which result in wide QRS complex and ECG findings of drop beat with bundle branch block pattern. The ratio of P to QRS is calculated as X:1 (2:1, 3:1 or 4:1) which indicates the number of P' wave that causes 1 QRS complex.

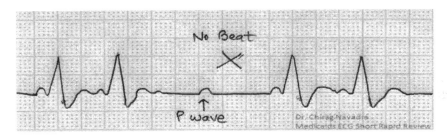

Figure 8.17: 2:1 AV block (QRS complex is generated after 2 P' waves)

CLINICAL PRESENTATION

- The patient is usually symptomatic and presents with palpitations, fatigue, dyspnea, chest pain, or light-headedness. Resulting bradycardia can compromise cardiac output and lead to hypotension, pallor, and syncope.
- Check if patient is taking any drugs such as beta-blockers, calcium blockers or digoxin that slow down the AV node.
- Check cardiac enzymes, potassium level and other perform other appropriate testing depending on suspected cause.
- 24-hour Holter monitoring and electrophysiological studies are indicated if the patient has developed syncope due to heart block.

MANAGEMENT

- **If the patient is asymptomatic:** no treatment
- **If the patient is symptomatic:** atropine is the drug of choice, epinephrine, dobutamine.
- **If the patient is symptomatic and atropine fail to control AV block**: Permanent pacing is the therapy of choice in advanced AV block. It does not require concomitant medical therapy.
- Temporary pacing is indicated as a bridging therapy for an emergency involving slow heart rate and for asystole caused by AV blocks.
- Discontinue digoxin, beta-blockers or calcium blockers if benefits outweigh the risk.
- If heart block is due to Lyme disease, add ceftriaxone.

3RD DEGREE AV BLOCK

- Complete AV block has defect anywhere from the inferior part of AV node to bundle branch purkinje system. AV dissociation is generally present in complete AV block where QRS complexes are conducted at their own rate and totally independent of the P wave.

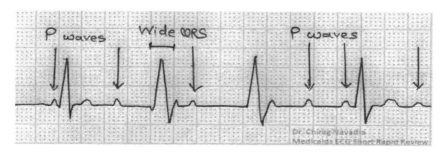

Figure 8.18: complete heart block

CLINICAL PRESENTATION

- The patient is usually symptomatic and hemodynamically unstable. Chief complaints include palpitations, fatigue, dyspnea, chest pain, or light-headedness. Resulting bradycardia can compromise cardiac output and lead to hypotension, pallor, and syncope.

Diagnostic workup and management is similar to Mobitz-type 2 AV block.

Permanent Pacing therapy:

- It is indicated in patient who present with syncope due to Mobitz type 2 AV block and complete heart block.
- Long term medication therapy along with permanent pacing therapy is not indicated.
- Acute complications of temporary or permanent pacing therapy include cardiac tamponade, hemothorax or pneumothorax.
- Infection of pacemaker or lead wire is rare and no prophylactic antibiotics are indicated.
- Patient is advised to restrict weight lifting for 4-6 weeks, and contact sports without wearing protective shield over the implanted pacemaker.

- There is a drop of beat but the cycle continues with normal rate and rhythm after a drop. It occurs due to block of electrical current from SA node to atria, thus no P' wave is present.

- In SA block, one entire ECG complex is absent and is multiple of R-R interval. Sinus arrest is when the pause is not a multiple of R-R interval. In other words, with SA block, the R-R interval measurement is within plus or minus 2 small boxes. If it is greater than 2 big boxes, it is sinus arrest.

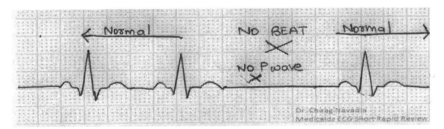

- SA blocks are generally asymptomatic and no treatment is required.

- If severe, it may cause fainting, altered mental status, chest pain, palpitations, dyspnea, hypoperfusion, and signs of shock.

- **Diagnosis:** in asymptomatic patient, no further workup is required. If symptomatic or an episode of syncope, 24-hour holter monitoring and exercise testing is indicated. Rule out electrolyte and thyroid abnormalities.

- **Treatment** - Not required for asymptomatic, but in emergent situation use atropine or transcutaneous pacing. If the patient is receiving medications that can provoke bradyarrhythmia, the medications should be stopped if possible.

RIGHT AND LEFT BUNDLE BRANCH BLOCKS

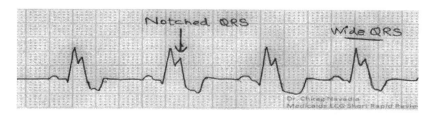

Bundle branch blocks are more commonly associated with coronary artery disease. It is a potential complication of myocardial infarction.

RIGHT BUNDLE BRANCH BLOCK

- Right bundle branch block (RBBB) is very common, and the risk of developing the condition increases with age. Once RBBB is identified on ECG, the next step is to rule out any underlying heart disease. RBBB is usually benign. No treatment is necessary in the patient with idiopathic RBBB and asymptomatic.
- If RBBB is symptomatic or associated with other heart conditions, such as an MI or other blocks in the electrical system, treatment is required accordingly. A pacemaker is required for bundle branch blocks.

Complete RBBB

- Wide QRS complex (>120ms)
- RSR' in leads V1 or V2. The R' deflection is usually wider than the initial R wave.
- S wave of greater duration than R wave or greater than 40ms in lead I and V6.

Incomplete RBBB

- Incomplete RBBB is defined by QRS duration between 110ms to 120ms in adults; other criteria are the same as for complete RBBB.
- The ECG pattern of incomplete RBBB may be present in the absence of other heart disease when r' is less than 20ms.
- In children, an RSR' pattern in V1 and V2 with a normal QRS duration is a normal variant.

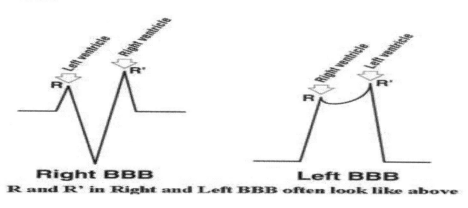

R and R' in Right and Left BBB often look like above

LEFT BUNDLE BRANCH BLOCK

- LBBBB are less common than RBBB and generally more severe in presentation than RBBB due to its effect on left ventricle. Due to slow conduction in LBBB, ventricular depolarization is delayed. The electrical activity in the left lateral wall is unopposed by right ventricular electrical activity. This causes left axis deviation.
- This block is usually caused by hypertensive heart disease, aortic stenosis, degenerative changes of the conduction system, myocarditis and coronary disease.
- Management is same like RBBB.

Complete LBBB

- Wide QRS complex (>120ms)

- Broad notched or slurred R waves in leads I, aVL, V5, and V6 and an occasional RS pattern in V5 and V6 attributed to displaced transition of QRS complex.

- Absent q waves in lateral leads I, V5, and V6, but in the lead aVL, a narrow q wave may be present in the absence of myocardial pathology.

- R-peak time >60ms in leads V5 and V6 but normal in leads V1, V2, and V3.

Incomplete LBBB

- QRS duration between 110ms and 119ms in adults. Other criteria are the same as for complete LBBB.
- Presence of left ventricular hypertrophy pattern.

When the QRS is wide and the definitions of LBBB and RBBB are not met, the term NIVCD (non-specific intraventricular conduction delay) is used.

Left anterior fascicular block: a condition that is distinguished from left bundle branch block by a defect in only the anterior half of the left bundle branch.

- It is the most common type of intraventricular conduction defect seen in acute anterior myocardial infarction.

- It can also be seen with acute inferior wall myocardial infarction, hypertensive heart disease, aortic valvular disease, and cardiomyopathies.

Left posterior fascicular block: a condition that is distinguished from left bundle branch block by a defect in only the posterior half of the left bundle branch.

The posterior half do not conduct impulse and so the electrical current goes through the other fascicle, and a frontal right axis deviation seen on the ECG.

BRUGADA SYNDROME

Brugada syndrome is an an autosomal dominant condition that causes disruption of heart's normal rhythm (specifically, ventricular arrhythmia) and sudden unexplained death in adults usually at night during sleep.

- It is more common in men of Asian ancestry (Japan, Thailand, and south-east Asia). The mean age of death due to ventricular fibrillation in Brugada syndrome is 40-years.

- Mutation in sodium channel gene is present in $1/3^{rd}$ of people with brugada syndrome. In other $2/3^{rd}$ of people, the cause is unknown.

- Family history of sudden death is usually present

Type 1	Type 2	Type 3
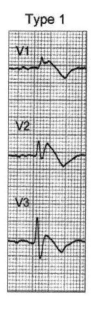	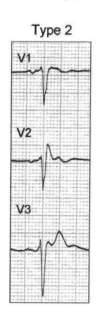	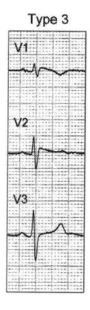

CLINICAL PRESENTATION

- Usually asymptomatic and often have family history of sudden cardiac death at age of 40 years.

- Syncope and sudden death is the most common clinical presentation

- Routine ECG might show ST elevation in V1-V3

- Associated with atrial fibrillation (20% cases)

DIAGNOSIS

- ECG is best initial test (done in all patient with syncope)

- Exclude other causes of syncope. Lab analysis to rule out hyperkalemia, hypercalcemia, cardiac enzymes and other potential causes of ST-segment elevation in right precordial leads.

- Echocardiography to rule out arrhythmogenic right ventricular cardiomyopathy and hypertrophic obstructive cardiomyopathy.

- Drug challenge with a sodium channel blocker in patients with syncope without an obvious cause.

- Genetic testing for SCN5 mutation (present in 1/3rd cases of Brugada syndrome.

MANAGEMENT

- Automatic implantable cardiac defibrillator (AICD) in symptomatic patient and abnormal electrophysiological study.

- If the patient is asymptomatic but has family history of Brugada syndrome, perform electrophysiological studies. If negative, routine follow up and no treatment is indicated.

- Drugs for long-term use are not recommended.

Although primary cardiac tumors are rare, they can be divided into:

- Benign (60-75% cases)
- Malignant (25-30% cases)

BENIGN TUMORS

Cardiac Myxoma

- Most common in adults
- Pedunculated mass in left atrium (most common location)
- Atrial myxoma can obstruct outflow from left atrium during diastole
- Asymptomatic if tumor is small
- Signs and symptoms of mitral stenosis occur with change in body positions like – breathing difficulty when lying flat, chest pain or tightness, dizziness, fainting, palpitations, shortness of breath with activity
- Surgery is the cure

Cardiac Lipoma – 10% cases of primary cardiac tumors. It is the second most common in adults. It is well-defined encapsulated mass of mature fat that contains few myocytes. Usually, lipomas are an incidental finding and rarely cause symptoms such as arrhythmias or obstruction, depending on their size and location. Asymptomatic lipomas: No treatment, symptomatic lipomas – resect it, good prognosis.

Cardiac Rhabdomyoma: most common primary cardiac tumor in children. It is of mesenchymal origin and associated with tuberous sclerosis. They are often multiple and located in left ventricle.

Papillary fibroelastosis – They are generally located on valves forming hair-like projections. As like cardiac myxoma, they arise from the endocardium and discovered incidentally. They have tendency to embolize systemically and therefore, surgery is indicated for large papillary fibroelastosis even in asymptomatic patient.

Other rare tumors:

- Cardiac hemangioma, pericardial teratoma (can rapidly grow despite being benign).

Cardiac Angiosarcoma

- Most common malignant primary cardiac tumor
- Tend to occur in right atrium
- More commonly involves pericardium

Rhabdomyosarcoma: rare, malignant tumor, affects the right side of the heart.

Pericardial mesothelioma:

- Associated with asbestos exposure
- A small intra-myocardial tumor that present with disturbances of the conduction system of the heart.
- Pericardiectomy to alleviate symptoms and chemotherapy to reduce tumor mass are commonly used palliative measures, however, prognosis is very poor.

Other rare tumors: primary cardiac osteosarcoma, malignant fibrous histiocytoma of heart, cardiac hemangiopericytoma, primary cardiac lymphoma

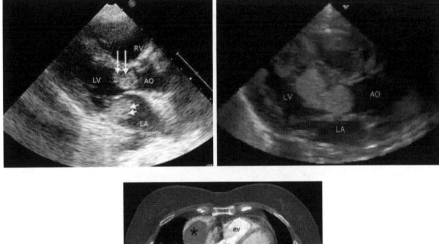

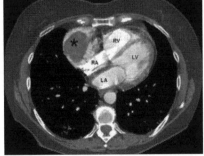

figure 9.1: cardiac myxoma*, **figure 9.2:** Rhabdomyoma*, **figure 9.3:** angiomyosarcoma*

ANTIARRHYTHMIC DRUGS

CLASS I: SODIUM CHANNEL BLOCKERS

Class IA antiarrhythmic

Drugs: Quinidine, Procainamide hydrochloride

- **Mechanism:** act on open or activated state Na+ channel of myocardium.

- Quinidine also blocks muscarinic and alpha receptors, so typical side effect caused by them is called as cinchonism (constipation/diarrhea, tinnitus, ocular dysfunction, CNS excitation, hypotension). It is never the first line drug for any arrhythmia but every medical exam loves to test on it.

- Procainamide: Less muscarinic block compared to quinidine, no alpha block. But, it acts like hapten, and adverse effect include drug-induced lupus in certain group of people who are slow acetylators, hematotoxicity, torsades rhythm. It is used in Wolf-Parkinson-White syndrome and acute ventricular arrhythmias.

- **Effect on ECG:** wide QRS complex and QT interval. No effect on SA/AV node.

Class IB antiarrhythmic

Drugs: Lidocaine hydrochloride

- **Mechanism:** blocks inactivated Na+ channel of myocardium, works best in hypoxic tissues

- **Effect on ECG:** decrease in QT interval, tachycardia, no effect on SA/AV node.

- **Use:** in acute ventricular arrhythmia, digoxin toxicity.

Class IC antiarrhythmic

Drugs: Flecainide, Propafenone

- **Mechanism:** blocks fast sodium channel, especially of His-Purkinje tissue.

- Highly pro-arrhythmogenic. Last choice drugs when all other option fails. Flecainide in combination with procainamide is used in Wolf-Parkinson-White syndrome.

- **Effect on ECG:** prolongs QRS, heart rate is variable.

CLASS II: BETA BLOCKERS

Drugs: metoprolol, acebutolol, propranolol, atenolol, esmolol and others.

- **Mechanism:** blocks beta-adrenergic receptors. they decrease SA and AV nodal activity, and increases diuresis.

- **Effect on ECG:** a small increase in PR interval and decrease in heart rate.

- **Use:** post-MI, angina (except Prinzmetal angina), hypertension, supraventricular tachycardia, thyrotoxicosis, migraine prophylaxis, anxiety.

  Propranolol is generally used for extra-cardiac manifestations such as thyrotoxicosis, and migraine prophylaxis.

  Esmolol is the beta-blocker of choice in emergency setting. It is not used for long-term management. Esmolol is used in acute supraventricular tachycardia, and hypertensive emergency.

  Carvedilol is a direct beta1 and alpha 1 blocker. It will have dual function of vasodilation along with decreases in heart rate.

- **Adverse effect:** bronchospasm, cold peripheries due to vasoconstriction (beta-2 block), fatigue, and hyperglycemia and sleep problems.

  B-blocker overdose will not lead to complete heart block but calcium channel blocker overdose can cause complete heart block.

- **Contraindication:** uncontrolled heart failure, severe asthma (mild asthma is not an absolute contraindication), sick sinus syndrome.

- Concurrent verapamil use may precipitate severe bradycardia and use of beta-blockers with verapamil is discouraged.

THUNDERNOTE

Theophylline

An end-line anti-asthmatic drug, which will cause bronchodilation by inhibiting phosphodiesterase and increasing cAMP level.

It will block the action of adenosine and higher dose of adenosine is required for adenosine testing in supraventricular tachycardia.

- B-Blockers can be used for theophylline-induced tachyarrhythmia.
- Barbiturates & Benzodiazepines can be used for theophylline-induced seizures.

CLASS III: POTASSIUM CHANNEL BLOCKERS

Drugs: amiodarone, sotalol, dofetilide

- Amiodarone: half-life is more than 80 days. Amiodarone has high tissue binding capacity and cytochrome P450 inhibitor. It increases concentration of digoxin and impairs the metabolism of warfarin, tending to potentiate its anticoagulant effect.

  It interferes with depolarization (class I antiarrhythmic), has beta blockade effect (class II antiarrhythmic), prolongs repolarization (class III antiarrhythmic), and has calcium channel blockade effect (class IV antiarrhythmic). It is the most effective antiarrhythmic for atrial fibrillation with structural heart disease, and symptomatic ventricular arrhythmias.

  Adverse effect: blue pigmentation of the skin, pulmonary fibrosis, corneal deposits, hepatotoxic, thyroid dysfunction, thrombophlebitis, peripheral neuropathy, prolongs QT interval (torsades).

- **Sotalol:** potassium channel and beta-blocker. Thus, sotalol decreases heart rate and decreases AV conduction also. The most salient feature of sotalol is its short half-life and acts quickly in life-threatening ventricular arrhythmias

CLASS IV: CALCIUM CHANNEL BLOCKERS

Drugs: verapamil, diltiazem (not used in hypertension management)

- **Mechanism:** blocks cardiac calcium channel in SA and AV node and decreases its electrical conductivity.

- **Adverse effect:** heart failure, constipation, hypotension, bradycardia

- **Use:** SVTs (supraventricular tachycardia), angina (other than prinzmetal angina)

- Beta blockers, verapamil and digoxin have additive AV nodal block effect. Combination of digoxin with beta-blockers is appropriate for low ejection fraction due to supraventricular arrhythmias or compensated heart failure, however combination of all 3 drugs is rarely indicated as there is high risk of AV nodal blockage.

Drugs: nifedipine, amlodipine

- **Mechanism:** blocks calcium channels in vasculature and act as a vasodilator. They will cause reflex tachycardia and can worsen angina due to increase in functionality of heart. Beta blockers are used to block this effect if necessary.

- **Use:** hypertension, prinzmetal angina and Reynauds phenomenon.

- Adverse effect: flushing, headache, ankle swelling, gingival hyperplasia [phenytoin and cyclosporine also increases risk of gingival hyperplasia in predisposed patients].

OTHER DRUGS

Adenosine

- **Mechanism:** decreases SA and AV nodal activity by decreasing cAMP (hyperpolarize the cell by potassium efflux). Duration of action is 10 seconds only.

- **Use:** It is used for both diagnosis and management of supraventricular tachycardia that do not improve with vagal maneuvers.

- **Drug interaction:** effects of adenosine is enhanced by dipyridamole, dopamine, and carbamazepine requiring lower dose of adenosine. Its effect is competitively blocked by theophylline and caffeine required higher dose of adenosine.

- **Adverse effect:** chest pain, **bronchospasm**, can enhance conduction down accessory pathways resulting in increased ventricular rate. Asthma, long QT syndrome, and 2nd or 3rd degree heart blocks are absolute contraindications.

Magnesium sulphate

- **Mechanism:** magnesium sulphate decrease the rate of SA node impulse generation, and prolongs the conduction time. It also stabilizes the excitatory membrane and blocks peripheral neuro-muscular transmission.

- **Use:** The first line drug for torsades-de-pointes (stabilizes the membrane), seizures in pregnancy.

- **Adverse effect:** respiratory depression, hypotension, reduced reflexes, hypothermia and pulmonary edema.

Digoxin

- **Mechanism:** digoxin is a cardiac glycoside that increases intracellular calcium by inhibiting cardiac Na-K+ ATPase. Digoxin will increase contractile force of the heart and block AV node by indirectly increasing vagal activity (by inhibiting neuronal Na-K+ ATPase).

- **Use:** congestive heart failure (for low ejection fraction), supraventricular tachycardia (except Wolf Parkinson White syndrome).

- Monitor potassium level when the patient is on digoxin (digoxin causes hyperkalemia.)

- **Adverse effect:** hyperkalemia, lethargy, nausea, vomiting, anorexia, confusion, visual disturbances, AV block when taken with beta-blockers or calcium channel blockers.

Drug interaction:

- Factors that increases toxicity of digoxin are **hypokalemia**, increasing age, renal failure, myocardial ischemia, hypomagnesemia, hypercalcemia, hypernatremia, hypoalbuminemia, hypothyroidism.
- Drugs such as amiodarone, quinidine, verapamil, diltiazem, spironolactone compete for secretion in distal convoluted tubule.
- Management of adverse effect: digibind (Fab antibodies toward digoxin) and supportive **electrolyte** therapy.

Atropine

- **Mechanism:** atropine is a competitive antagonist at muscarinic acetylcholine receptor. It dilates the pupils, increases heart rate and reduces secretions such as lacrimation and salivation.

- **Use:** sinus bradycardia, asystole or pulseless electrical activity, organophosphate poisoning.

- **Adverse effect:** tachyarrhythmia, precipitates narrow-angle glaucoma, dry mouth.

ANTIHYPERTENSIVE DRUGS

Beta Blockers and calcium channel blockers are discussed earlier in anti-arrhythmic section.

VASODILATORS

Epinephrine

- **Mechanism:** Epinephrine has effect on beta-1, beta-2 and alpha-1 action.

  Low dose: increases heart rate and vasodilation due to beta-1 and beta-2 effects.

  Medium dose: increases heart rate only due to beta-1 action. Beta-2 causes vasodilation and alpha causes vasoconstriction and so, their effect will be nullified.

  High dose: alpha 1 action predominates, thereby increasing total peripheral resistance and blood pressure.

- **Use:** anaphylactic shock (drug of choice), cardiac arrest

- **Adverse effects:** tachyarrhythmia, anxiety, tremors, severe hypertension or cerebral hemorrhage if given with non-selective beta-blockers (beta action cancels out, alpha action predominates)

Nesiritide

- **Mechanism:** nesiritide is a recombinant form of the human beta-type natriuretic peptide. The natriuretic peptide is released from ventricular myocytes in response to an increase in blood volume and atrial pressure. Nesiritide cause generalized vascular relaxation and decrease Na+ reabsorption in the medullary collecting tubule. It constricts efferent renal arterioles and dilates afferent arterioles (cGMP-mediated).

- It has mild diuretic effects and contributing to the "escape from aldosterone" mechanism.

- **Use:** it is never the first line or even second line drug for any condition. It can be use in decompensated congestive heart failure but no evidence showing that Nesiritide can lower mortality.

NITRATES

Drugs: isosorbide dinitrate, nitroprusside, nitroglycerin

- **Mechanism:** nitric oxide mediated vasodilation effects to reduce both preload and afterload. It has predominant effect on the veins thereby, decreasing preload and work load (oxygen demand) of the heart. It also dilates the coronary arteries.

- **Use:** anginal attacks, acute treatment of heart failure.

Sublingual nitroglycerin is the most common drug used in patients to relieve angina attacks by venodilation. Nitroglycerin decreases symptoms of acute MI but does not decrease mortality. Isosorbide dinitrate can be use in hypertensive emergencies.

- **Adverse effect:** hypotension, tachycardia, headaches and rarely prolong infusion can cause **methemoglobinemia.**

- **Contraindication:** recent use of PDE-V inhibitors such as sildenafil in last 24 hours, hypotension, shock. Avoid use in hypertrophic cardiomyopathy or aortic stenosis where decreasing preload can worsen the condition.

ACE-INHIBITORS

Drugs: enalapril, lisinopril, captopril, ramipril

- **Mechanism**: ACE-inhibitors act by inhibiting the conversion angiotensin I to angiotensin II in lungs. Angiotensin II is a potent vasoconstrictor and cause sodium-water retention via aldosterone.

- **Use**: hypertension (young, diabetics), heart failure, diabetic nephropathy.

- **Adverse effect:** cough (due to increase in bradykinin levels in the lungs), angioedema, hyperkalemia (because of decreased aldosterone), first-dose hypotension (more common in patients taking diuretics)

- **Contraindication:** pregnancy and breastfeeding (class IV drug), **bilateral** renal artery stenosis, aortic stenosis (may result in hypotension, hereditary of idiopathic angioedema

- **Precaution:** urea and electrolytes level should be checked before treatment is initiated. Rise in creatinine and potassium is expected after starting ACE inhibitors. Acceptable changes are an increase in serum creatinine, up to 30% from baseline

ANGIOTENSIN RECEPTOR BLOCKERS

Drugs: losartan, candesartan, and valsartan

Mechanism: ARBs blocks the angiotensin receptors and therefore, no pulmonary adverse effect. Although, ACE-inhibitors and ARBs have similar action, receptors get desensitized when any receptor blocker drugs are used for long period of time and therefore ACE-inhibitors are generally preferred before ARBs for chronic management.

Use: ARBs are used when patient develop 'cough' due to ACE inhibitor. If the patient has hyperkalemia due to ACE inhibitor, ARBs are not indicated

Hydralazine

- **Mechanism:** hydralazine is a direct acting vasodilator. It has predominant effect on the arterioles reducing total peripheral resistance. It acts by increasing cGMP leading to arterial smooth muscle relaxation

- **Use:** hypertension in pregnancy, hypertensive crisis.

- **Adverse effect:** hypotension, palpitations, flushing, fluid retention, headache, drug-induced lupus.

- **Contraindication:** Drug induced-SLE, coronary artery disease (coronary still phenomenon) and rheumatic valve disease (mitral stenosis).

DIURETICS

Loop diuretics: furosemide, bumetanide

- **Mechanism:** inhibits the Na-K-Cl transporter in the thick ascending limb of the loop of Henle, reducing the reabsorption of sodium and water. Aldosterone mediated sodium reabsorption is increased at distal tubules and thereby, it causes mild hypokalemia.

- **Use:** first line drug for isolated hypertension, volume overload cardiac condition such as heart failure (use intravenously for acute heart failure, use orally for chronic), and resistant hypertension particularly in patients with renal impairment.

- **Adverse effect:** hypotension, hyponatremia, hypokalemia, hypochloremic alkalosis, ototoxicity (ethacrynic acid is most toxic), hypocalcemia, renal impairment (due to dehydration + direct toxic effect), hyperglycemia (less common than with thiazides), gout.

Thiazides: hydrochlorothiazide

- **Mechanism:** inhibit Na+/Cl- transporter on distal tubules. This will increase calcium reabsorption in expense of sodium reabsorption.

- **Use:** hypertension, heart failure, **nephrolithiasis** (calcium stones), nephrogenic diabetic insipedus.

- **Adverse effect:** sulfonamide hypersensitivity, hypokalemic alkalosis, hypercalcemia, **hyperuricemia, hyperglycemia,** hyperlipidemia.

- **Contraindication:** sulphonamide hypersensitivity. Although they are not absolutely contraindicated in diabetes or gout, care should be taken while prescribing in such patients.

Potassium-sparing diuretics

Drugs: spironolactone, amiloride, triamterene

Spironolactone

- **Mechanism:** aldosterone receptor antagonist on collecting ducts of kidney.

- **Use:** hyperaldosteronism, adjunct to potassium wasting diuretics, antiandrogenic use, congestive heart failure

- **Adverse effect:** hyperkalemic acidosis, anti-androgenic effects (gynecomastia in males, hirsutism, acne in female)

Amiloride and Triamterene

- **Mechanism:** sodium channel blocker on collecting ducts of kidney.

- **Use:** adjunct to loops or thiazide diuretics, lithium-induced diabetes insipedus.

- **Adverse effect:** hyperkalemic acidosis.

Carbonic anhydrase inhibitors (acetazolamide, dorzolamide)

- **Mechanism:** carbonic anhydrase inhibitor and has organ specific activity. In the eye, it decreases the rate of aqueous humor production and decreases intraocular pressure. In the kidney, it inhibits H^+ ion excretion and decreases sodium reabsorption (mild effect). Electrolyte changes that can occur are hypokalemia (little amount of sodium is reabsorbed in exchange of potassium ions) and acidosis (due to bicarbonate loss in urine and H^+ retention).

- **Use:** congestive heart failure, glaucoma, acute mountain sickness, metabolic alkalosis

- **Contraindication:** hypokalemia, hyperchloremic acidosis, liver cirrhosis

Osmotic diuretics (mannitol)

- **Use:** glaucoma (to decrease intraocular pressure), cerebral edema, Oliguric states (Rhabdomyolysis), bronchiectasis (for clearance of mucus). It is not use for any cardiac-related problem.

- **Adverse effect: Pulmonary edema**

Ranolazine

- **Mechanism:** inhibits late sodium cardiac current that reduces intracellular calcium.

- **Use:** Recently, approved for management of chronic stable angina. It is used in combination with other anti-anginal drugs who are not responsive to maximally tolerated doses of other standard antianginal medications. It is not used for acute anginal attacks and NSTEMI

- **Adverse effects:** dizziness, nausea, vomiting, constipation, prolongs QT interval (risk of torsade de pointes)

- **Contraindication:** liver disease and cytochrome P450 inhibitors decreases its clearance from the liver.

Atherosclerosis is often associated with hypercholesterolemia.

STATINS

Drugs: atorvastatin, lovastatin, -statin

- **Mechanism: statins** inhibit HMG-CoA reductase enzyme in the liver. This will decrease liver cholesterol production and increase in LDL receptor expression for LDL endocytosis. They also mildly decrease triglyceride synthesis and increases HDL level.

- **Use:** maximum benefits are observed in individual with clinical acute coronary syndrome, isolated LDL >190 mg/dl, individual with diabetes and age >75 years.

- **Adverse effect:** myalgia, rhabdomyolysis, hepatotoxic. Increase risk of rhabdomyolysis if combined with gemfibrozil (antihyperlipidemic that decreases triglyceride level).

BILE ACID SEQUESTRANTS

- **Drug:** cholestyramine

- **Mechanism:** cholestyramine binds to the bile salts in the gut and prevents reabsorption through intestine. This will decrease enterohepatic circulation of bile salts and circulating LDL. Statins are still the best drug to lower LDL.

- **Adverse effect:** mal-absorption of lipid soluble vitamins leads to vitamin A, D, E and K deficiency over the period of time, increases VLDL and triglyceride level.

- **Contraindication:** hypertriglyceridemia, complete biliary obstruction. Cautions should be taken if the patient is volume depleted or has renal impairement.

NIACIN

- **Mechanism:** niacin is a component of enzymes necessary for lipid metabolism, glycogenolysis, inhibits synthesis of VLDL and increases synthesis of HDL.

- **Adverse effect:** flushing, itching and stomach upset. Control adverse effects such as flushing by using aspirin before taking niacin.

- **Use:** It is not primarily used for lowering LDL but are used for increasing HDL levels as adjuvant therapy for mixed dyslipidemia.

Gemfibrozil

- **Mechanism:** gemfibrozil is an activator of peroxisome proliferator-activated receptors (PPAR) that induces production of lipoprotein lipases and decreases VLDL, LDL.

- **Use:** hypertriglyceridemia, not used for hypocholesteremia.

- **Adverse effect:** gallstone, myositis (when taken in combination with statins), thromboembolism

Ezetimibe

- **Mechanism:** prevent intestinal absorption of cholesterol and thus decreases LDL.

- No clinical trial had shown that ezetimibe reduced heart attack, stroke or death. AHA does not recommend ezetimibe, however, it can be used as a second line to those who are unable to achieve target LDL cholesterol levels on statins alone.

Omega-3 Fatty Acid Ethyl Esters

- Derived from fish oils. Intended to be used in addition to diet to lower very high triglyceride (levels over 500 mg/dL).
- **Adverse effect:** cough, difficulty swallowing, dizziness, tachycardia, itching, puffiness around eyes, chest discomfort.

ANTICOAGULANTS

Anticoagulants reduce blood clotting. This prevents deep vein thrombosis, pulmonary embolization, systemic embolization, and myocardial infarction.

Heparin

- Heparin works by activating antithrombin III which blocks thrombin and prevent formation of clot.

- **Unfractionated heparin:** equal activity against factor Xa and factor IIa (thrombin). Highest risk of heparin induced thrombocytopenia.

- **Enoxaparin** is a Low molecular weight heparin that binds more to Factor IIa only and has less antithrombotic activity compared to unfractionated heparin. LMWH is most commonly preferred heparin. Although, heparin induced thrombocytopenia is less common with LMWH, it should not be used in heparin-induced thrombocytopenia.

- Rivaroxaban, apixaban, edoxaban are **factor Xa Inhibitor.**

- Lepirudin, bivalirudin, dabigatran, ximelagatran are direct **factor IIa Inhibitor.**

Complication: Heparin Induced Thrombocytopenia; 2 types

- **Type I:** develops in first 2 days after the exposure to heparin. It is due to the direct effect of heparin on platelet activation. Type 1 HIT is not severe enough to cause thrombotic complications.

- **Type II:** develops 4-10 days after exposure to heparin. It is immune-mediated (antibodies againts platelet factor-4) and has severe life **threatening prothrombotic complications**. HIT must be suspected if patient receiving heparin therapy has a 50% fall in platelets count. Venous thrombosis is more common than arterial thrombosis.

Serotonin release assay is the confirmatory test but If heparin induced thrombocytopenia is suspected, heparin must be stopped immediately. Switch the patient to other direct factor inhibitors such as argatroban or lepirudin. Argatroban is not indicated in patient with liver cirrhosis because it is cleared by liver. Lepirudin is not indicated in patient with chronic renal failure because it is cleared by kidneys.

Warfarin

- Warfarin inhibits vitamin K epoxide reductase (prevent gamma-carboxylation which is necessary for vitamin K function)

- It takes at least 48 to 72 hours for the anticoagulant effect to develop and therefore heparin must be given concomitantly for first few days.

- Warfarin is contraindicated in pregnancy during first trimester (low molecular weight heparin is indicated)

Complication

- Thrombotic (warfarin skin necrosis) on day 3-7

- Bleeding occurs on day 10 onwards. High risk of bleeding in elderly people.

- **Warfarin skin necrosis:** warfarin works by inactivating vitamin K dependent clotting factors II, VII, IX, X, C & S. Protein C and S are natural anticoagulants with short half-life while factor II, VII, IX and X has longer half-life. Although rare, when warfarin is given, protein C and S will be deficient before coagulating factors and therefore, high risk of thrombosis. Heparin is given for first 4-5 days to prevent such complication.

  Histopathology of warfarin necrosis usually reveals clotting within blood vessels in the skin without any inflammation.

  Warfarin can also precipitate calciphylaxis, recognized on biopsy by calcium deposition in the affected skin.

  Warfarin skin necrosis is seen more commonly in patient with hereditary deficiency of protein C and protein S. Therefore, if the patient develops warfarin skin necrosis, first step in management is to check protein C and protein S levels. It is rare and routine testing is not recommended. The mainstay of treatment is to stop warfarin. If anticoagulation is required, heparin can be used.

- In acute bleeding, fresh frozen plasma is used for reversal of warfarin induced bleeding.

Recently FDA approved Prothrombin Complex Concentrate (Kcentra) for urgent reversal of warfarin mediated coagulation factor deficiency with acute major bleeding (not indicated in patients without bleeding due to potential for thromboembolic complications). Fresh frozen plasma is still the most preferred choice for warfarin related bleeding.

FIBRINOLYTICS

Tissue Plasminogen Activator (alteplase, reteplase)

- TPA converts plasminogen to plasmin. Plasmin will chop off the formed fibrin clot. It does not help in clot prevention.
- **Use:** pulmonary embolism, myocardial infarction and ischemic stroke (administered as early as possible.
- **Adverse effect:** severe hemorrhage.
- **Contraindication:** stroke in last 3-6 months, intracranial hemorrhage at any time, head injury in last 3 months, known history of arteriovenous malformation, brain tumor or active bleeding.

Urokinase

- It is similar to tPA. In fact, it has quicker action than tPA but very costly and therefore, tPA is more commonly preferred.

- Shortened lysis time indicates a hyper-fibrinolytic state and bleeding risk with tPA. Hyper-fibrinolytic state includes liver disease, plasminogen activator inhibitor deficiency or alpha-2 antiplasmin deficiency.

NON-PHARMACOLOGICAL MANAGEMENT

Lifestyle modification: elimination of caffeine, alcohol, or any other substances believed to be causing the problem, stress-reduction measures, such as meditation, stress management classes, an exercise program, or psychotherapy.

Cardioversion: In this procedure, an electrical shock is delivered to the heart through the chest to stop certain very fast arrhythmias such as atrial fibrillation, supraventricular tachycardia, or atrial flutter. The patient is connected to an ECG monitor, which is also connected to the defibrillator. **Cardioversion** is a synchronized administration of shock during the R waves or QRS complex of a cardiac cycle. **Defibrillation** is a non-synchronized random administration of shock during a cardiac cycle.

It causes all of the heart cells to contract simultaneously. This interrupts and terminates abnormal electrical rhythm. This, in turn, allows the sinus node to resume normal pacemaker activity. They are contraindicated in dysrhythmias due to enhanced automaticity such as digitalis toxicity, multifocal atrial tachycardia. If performed, life threatening ventricular arrhythmias can occur.

Defibrillation and cardioversion are also ineffective in asystole because they terminate abnormal electrical rhythm and allow time for SA for resume normal activity. In asystole, there is no normal or abnormal rhythm. Perform CPR and give epinephrine.

Ablation: This is an invasive procedure done in the electrophysiology laboratory, which means that a catheter is inserted into the heart through a vessel in the groin or arm. The procedure is done in a manner similar to the electrophysiology studies (EPS). Once the site of the arrhythmia has been determined by EPS, the catheter is moved to the site. By use of a technique, such as radiofrequency ablation (very high frequency radio waves are applied to the site, heating the tissue until the site is destroyed) or cryoablation (an ultra-cold substance is applied to the site, freezing the tissue and destroying the site), the site of the arrhythmia may be destroyed.

Pacemaker: permanent pacemaker is a small device that is implanted under the skin (most often in the shoulder area just under the collar bone), and sends electrical signals to start or regulate a slow heartbeat. A permanent pacemaker may be used to make the heart beat if the heart's natural pacemaker (the SA node) is not functioning properly and has developed an abnormal heart rate or rhythm or if the electrical pathways are blocked. Pacemakers are typically used for slow arrhythmias such as sinus bradycardia, sick sinus syndrome, or heart block.

Implantable cardioverter defibrillator: An implantable cardioverter defibrillator (ICD) is a small device, similar to a pacemaker that is implanted under the skin, often in the shoulder area just under the collarbone. An ICD senses the rate of the heartbeat. When the heart rate exceeds a rate programmed into the device, it delivers an electrical shock to the heart in order to correct the rhythm to a slower more normal heart rhythm. ICDs are combined with a pacemaker to deliver an electrical signal to regulate a heart rate that is too slow. ICDs are used for life-threatening fast arrhythmias such as ventricular tachycardia or ventricular fibrillation.

Surgery: surgical treatment for arrhythmias is usually done only when all other appropriate options have failed. Surgical ablation is a major surgical procedure requiring general anesthesia. The chest is opened, exposing the heart. The site of the arrhythmia is located; the tissue is destroyed or removed in order to eliminate the source of the arrhythmia.

CONGRATULATIONS

YOU ARE READY TO SCORE MAXIMUM ON YOUR BOARDS

TODAY YOU LEARNT SOMETHING THAT YOUR COLLEAGUES MIGHT NOT KNOW

YOU ACCOMPLISHED AN ACHIEVEMENT THAT YOU RIGHTLY DESERVED

BE PROUD OF CARDIOLOGY GURU

Along with this book, I would also recommend you to do some clinical cases from your preferred question bank and you will be a rock-star during your rotations or patient care.

If you have android phone, we have over 200+ Free USMLE cases in our free app: USMLE CASE CHALLENGE. One case is posted everyday day to decrease your fatigue level. Solve it before you go to sleep or when you wake up.

But for now, I just hope that this book has not disappointed you. If you feel that "Fundamental of Cardiology" is not worth for you, kindly contact us within 14 days of your purchase to receive your partial refund.

www.medrx-education.com

"Let the smile be your and your patient's umbrella" – Chirag N

Please, please, please give me 2 minutes and rate 'fundamentals of cardiology' on amazon. Send me any suggestion that you would like to improve in future editions.

THANKS FOR BELIEVING IN ME AND MY BOOK

I wish you all a very happy, peaceful medical practice and of course, a cheerful life.

CHIRAG NAVADIA, MD

WORLD CLASS TRUSTED REFERENCES

- Guidelines for valvular pathology, 2014
  http://content.onlinejacc.org/article.aspx?articleid=1838843

- http://qjmed.oxfordjournals.org/content/102/4/235.full

- Pericardial disease, Guidelines
  http://www.ncbi.nlm.nih.gov/pmc/articles/PMC2878263/#!po=1.19048

- Naxos disease, http://circ.ahajournals.org/content/116/20/e524.full

- http://www.merckmanuals.com/professional/cardiovascular_disorders/cardiovascular_tests_
  and_procedures/percutaneous_coronary_interventions_pci.html

- HOCM Guidelines, 2011, http://content.onlinejacc.org/article.aspx?articleid=1147838

- Infective Endocarditis, http://emedicine.medscape.com/article/216650-overview\

- Guidelines of stable IHD, 2014 http://content.onlinejacc.org/article.aspx?marticleid=1891717

- http://emedicine.medscape.com/article/892980-treatment#aw2aab6b6b3

- Management of Deep venous thrombosis and PE, 2012 ACCP Guidelines,
  http://professionalsblog.clotconnect.org/2012/02/27/new-accp-guidelines-%E2%80%93-dvt-
  and-pe-highlights-and-summary/

- http://circ.ahajournals.org/content/122/18_suppl_3/S829.full
- http://eurheartj.oxfordjournals.org/content/32/24/3147.full
- Jugulovenous pressure, http://www.ncbi.nlm.nih.gov/books/NBK300/
- Katranci AO, Görk AS, Rizalar R et al. (2012). "Pentalogy of Cantrell". Indian J Pediatr 65
  (1): 149–53.
- http://www.nejm.org/cardiology
- http://content.onlinejacc.org/article.aspx?articleid=1188032
- Carvajal syndrome, http://circ.ahajournals.org/content/116/20/e524.full
- Rapid Review of Pathology, 4th Edition, Edward Goljan
- Robins and Contran pathology, Basis of disease, 9e, Vinay Kumar, Abul k. Abbas Jon C
  Aster,
- Master the Boards, Internal Medicine, Conrad Fischer, http://www.mastertheboards.com/
- Guidelines on SVT & VT http://content.onlinejacc.org/article.aspx?articleid=1132718
- http://www.ncbi.nlm.nih.gov/pubmed/1880230
- http://www.healio.com/cardiology
- http://www.ncbi.nlm.nih.gov/pubmed/11673357
- http://www.merckmanuals.com/professional
- www.openi.nlm.nih.gov/detailedresult.php?img=2856576_vhrm-6-207f2&req=4

No content from the above sources is directly copied in this book. No laws were broken. These are just some efforts to make this book most updated cardiology book according to the guidelines. However, nobody is perfect and we want you to make this book 99% accurate by sending us any new updates or mistakes.

IMAGE CREDENTIALS

Figure 1.4: septum development of the atrium, **www.nature.com**

Figure 1.5: septum development of the ventricles, **www.memorize.com**

Figure 2.1: chest x-ray, widened mediastinum, **www.wikipedia.org**

Figure 2.2: CT at T4, : **www.aboutcancer.com**

Figure 2.3: CT at T5, **www.meddean.luc.edu**

Figure 2.4: mediastinal mass Image source - **www.escholarship.org**

Figure 2.7: frontal view of the chest cavity on chest x-ray, University of Auckland

Figure 2.8: atrial and ventricular pacemaker spike, **www.medrx-education.com**

Figure 2.10: territories of coronary arteries, Principles of anatomy and physiology 11e John Wiley & Sons

Figure 3.2: vascular diameter, cross-section area, blood pressure and velocity of blood flow, **www.cnx.org**

Figure 3.5: pulmonary pressure curve, **Figure 3.6:** pulse pressure change, **www.medrx-education.com**

Figure 3.7: performance change with increase in preload and contractility, **www.medrx-education.com**

Figure 3.8: effects of preload, afterload, contractility and heart rate, **www.medrx-education.com**

Figure 3.9: effect of vasoconstrictors, **Figure 3.10:** effect of change in volume, **www.medrx-education.com**

Figure 3.11: action potential in fast fibers **Figure 3.12:** in slow response fibers, **www.medrx-education.com**

Figure 3.22: systolic and diastolic murmurs, **www.wikipedia.org**

Figure 3.23: jugular venous pressure waves in various valvular pathology, **www.rjmatthewsmd.com**

Figure 4.2: subarachnoid hemorrhage, www.cdemcurriculum.org/

Figure 4.3: hyaline Arteriolosclerosis, **www.missinglink.ucsf.edu**

Figure 4.4: hyperplastic Arteriolosclerosis, **www.web.squ.edu.om/**

Figure 4.10: thoracic aortic aneurysm, www.cardiophile.com

Figure 4.11: abdominal aortic aneurysm, **www.lumen.luc.edu**

Figure 4.14: CT showing aortic dissection, **Figure 4.15:** types of aortic dissection, **www.wikipedia.org**

Figure 4.16: right-sided multiple rib fractures and flail chest, www.trauma.org/

Figure 4.17: rib notching (bilateral red arrows), www.radiographia.ru

Figure 4.18: MRA showing coarctation of aorta, **www.medglobus.ru**

Figure 4.19: angiogram of polyarteritis nodosa, **www.wikipedia.org**

Figure 4.20: Takayasu arteritis, www.hopkinsvasculitis.org/

Figure 4.21: pallor, cyanosis, **Figure 5.1:** venous system, **Figure 5.4:** swelling in leg, www.wikipedia.org

Figure 5.5: pitting edema due to CHF (bilateral), **www.byebyedoctor.com**

Figure 6.2: muscle rupture **Figure 6.3:** ventricular aneurysm **Figure 6.4:** scar tissue, **www.wikipedia.org**

Figure 6.5: coronary arteries and 12-leads, **www.slideshare.net**

Figure 6.6: inferior wall MI, James Heilman, MD, **www.wikipedia.org**

Figure 6.8: lateral wall MI, **www.lifeinthefastlane.com**

Figure 6.9: Coronary angiogram, Melhem et al. Thrombosis Journal 2009 7:5

Figure 6.11: diastole. Salim Virani, MD, Texas Heart Institute

Figure 6.12: echocardiogram in dilated cardiomyopathy, **Figure 6.13:** enlarged globular heart on chest x-ray, **Figure 6.14:** right and left ventricle walls are severely thickened, **www.wikipedia.org**

Figure 6.16: concentric hypertrophy, **peir.path.uab.edu**

Figure 6.19: RV dilation, **Figure 6.21:** Diffuse ST elevation, **Figure 6.22:** calcification, www.wikipedia.org

Figure 6.23: white calcific line surrounding the heart), www.radiopedia.org

Figure 6.24: fibrinous pericarditis

Figure 6.26: pericardial effusion, www.onlinejets.org/

Figure 6.26: massive cardiomegaly, www.jaypeejournals.com/

Figure 6.28: large vegetations of infective endocarditis, heart.bmj.com/

Figure 6.29: small vegetations of NBTE www.revespcardiol.org/

Figure 6.30: Osler node, **figure 6.31:** splinter hemorrhage, www.wikipedia.org

Figure 6.32: Roth spots, www.aao.org/

Figure 6.33: bicuspid aortic stenosis, www.health-writings.com/

Figure 6.36: Aschoff nodule, Dr. Edwin Ewing

Figure 8.1: Atrioventricular nodal re-entrant tachycardia, Dr. Lorenzo

Figure 8.7: proptosis, **Figure 8.14:** peak T-wave, www.wikipedia.org

UPDATES

If you find anything incorrect or aware of new future updates, please note it down on this page and send it to us. Your efforts will not be worthless. If your suggestions are included in our next edition, you will be given a special acknowledgment in the beginning of our book

BEST WISHES FROM THE DEPTH OF MARIANA TRENCH